RESPIRATORY MANAGEMENT OF NEWBORNS

Edited by **Hany Aly**
and **Hesham Abdel-Hady**

Respiratory Management of Newborns
http://dx.doi.org/10.5772/61451
Edited by Hany Aly and Hesham Abdel-Hady

Contributors
Joanne Baerg, Arul Thirumoorthi, Andrew Hopper, Alejandro G Gonzalez-Garay, Vicente Gonzalez-Bustamante, Guilherme Sant'Anna, Wissam Shalish, Georg Schmolzer, Anne Solevag, Po-Yin Cheung, Megan O'Reilly, Pia Wintermark, Asim Al Balushi, Maria Agustina Lopez Laporte, Leif Nelin, Edward Shepherd, Susan Lynch, Daniel Malleske, Begum Atasay, Martin Francis Joyce-Brady, Lou Ann Scism Brown, Petja Fister, Štefan Grosek

Published by InTech
Janeza Trdine 9, 51000 Rijeka, Croatia

Publishing Process Manager Edi Lipovic
Technical Editor SPi Global
Cover InTech Design team

First published August, 2016
Printed in Croatia

Additional hard copies can be obtained from orders@intechopen.com

Respiratory Management of Newborns, Edited by Hany Aly and Hesham Abdel-Hady
p. cm.
Print ISBN 978-953-51-2574-7
Online ISBN 978-953-51-2575-4

Meet the editors

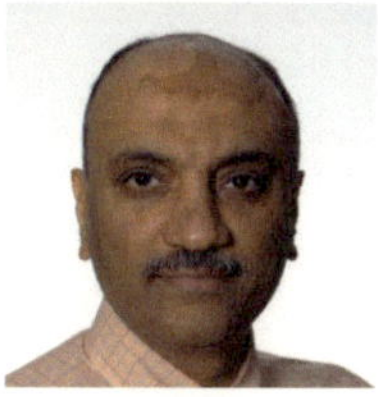

Dr. Hany Aly is a professor in Pediatrics and Obstetrics at the George Washington University and Children's National Medical Center. He is the director of the Division of Newborn Services at the George Washington University Medical Center in Washington, DC, USA, and the editor-in-chief for *Journal of Neonatal-Perinatal Medicine*. He is a regional trainer for the Neonatal Resuscitation and a member of the American Academy of Pediatrics, American Pediatric Society, and Society of Pediatric Research.

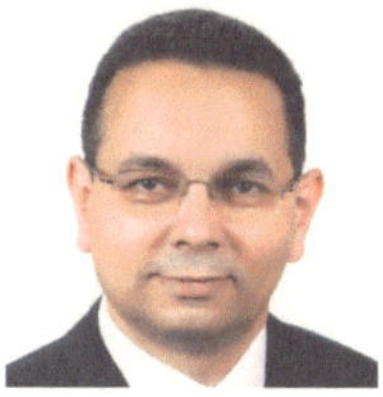

Dr. Hesham Abdel-hady is a professor in Pediatric/Neonatology and Chief of the Division of Neonatology at Mansoura University Children's Hospital in Egypt. He is a regional trainer for the Neonatal Resuscitation Program of the American Academy of Pediatrics, a board member of the International Society for Evidence-Based Neonatology (EBNEO), a member of the Society of Pediatric Research, and an editorial board member for multiple international journals.

Contents

Preface IX

Chapter 1 **Respiratory Function During Chest Compressions 1**
Georg M Schmölzer, Anne Solevåg, Erica McGinn, Megan O'Reilly and Po-Yin Cheung

Chapter 2 **Alternative Therapies for the Management of Respiratory Distress Syndrome 11**
Alejandro González-Garay and Vicente González-Bustamante

Chapter 3 **Respiratory Management of the Newborn with an Omphalocele 25**
Joanne Baerg, Arul Thirumoorthi and Andrew Hopper

Chapter 4 **Respiratory Care Protocols in Neonatal Intensive Care 51**
Wissam Shalish and Guilherme Mendes Sant' Anna

Chapter 5 **The Impact of Ventilation on the Development of Brain Injury in Asphyxiated Newborns Treated with Hypothermia 71**
Asim Al Balushi, Maria A. Lopez Laporte and Pia Wintermark

Chapter 6 **Mechanical Ventilation of the Infant with Severe Bronchopulmonary Dysplasia 83**
Edward G. Shepherd, Susan K. Lynch, Daniel T. Malleske and Leif D. Nelin

Chapter 7 **Respiratory Distress and Management Strategies in the Newborn 95**
Begüm Atasay, İlke Mungan Akın and Serdar Alan

Chapter 8 **Perinatal Lung Development: The Lung at Birth 119**
Jyh-Chang Jean, Lou Ann Scism Brown and Martin Joyce-Brady

Chapter 9 **Non-Pulmonary Management of Newborns with Respiratory Distress 139**
Petja Fister and Štefan Grosek

Preface

Respiratory management of the newborn is a broad field in which we are convinced it is hard to be efficiently covered in a single book; therefore, we did not intend to cover the basic knowledge and the day-to-day routine management of infants with respiratory distress. Readers can easily find such information in various sources. The scope of this book is to focus on a few specific areas of respiratory management that are often challenging. For example, it covers ventilator management of infants with unusually severe bronchopulmonary dysplasia and infants with omphalocele. The book also provides an overview on new trends in the management of fetal and transitioning lungs in infants delivered prematurely, positioning of endotracheal tube in extremely low birth weight infants, noninvasive respiratory support, and utilization of a strategy stems on protocol-driven respiratory management.

Neonatal resuscitation is a cornerstone skill for healthcare providers in the field of neonatology. The interest to ensure efficacious resuscitation and to monitor physiologic parameters of neonates during chest compression cannot be overemphasized. This book includes a chapter on noninvasive respiratory function monitoring during chest compression analyzing the efficacy and quality of chest compression and exhaled carbon dioxide.

Lastly, the relationship between ventilator-related lung injury and brain development is an area of recent interest; we like to use the term "lung-brain axis," and we believe there is a wealth of knowledge yet to be discovered in this area of management. This book includes a chapter on neonatal encephalopathy treated with hypothermia along with mechanical ventilation. The interaction of cooling with respiration and the strategies to optimize oxygenation and ventilation in asphyxiated newborns are discussed. This book brings new information in a simplified structure that allows readers to enjoy as they learn. We thank contributing authors for their valuable time and expertise that made this book possible.

Hany Aly, MD, FAAP
The George Washington University and the Children's National Medical Center
Washington, DC, USA

Hesham Abdel-Hady, MD
Mansoura University Children's Hospital
Mansoura, Egypt

Chapter 1

Respiratory Function During Chest Compressions

Georg M Schmölzer, Anne Solevåg, Erica McGinn,
Megan O'Reilly and Po-Yin Cheung

Additional information is available at the end of the chapter

http://dx.doi.org/10.5772/63510

Abstract

Chest compression (CC) is an infrequent event (0.08%) in newborns delivered at near-term and term gestation, and occurs at a higher frequency (10%) in preterm deliveries. In addition, outcome studies of deliveries requiring resuscitation or chest compression have reported high rates of mortality and neurodevelopmental impairment in surviving children. A respiratory function monitor (RFM) can help guide a resuscitator during cardiopulmonary resuscitation (CPR) in a neonate and help assess the quality and efficacy of chest compression. Utilizing a non-invasive respiratory function monitor during chest compression may decrease high mortality rates in addition to having many distinct advantages, which will benefit both the newborn and the resuscitators. There are several different ways that a respiratory function monitor can assist a resuscitator during chest compression; these include confirming and ensuring adequate lung ventilation, analyzing the efficacy and quality of chest compression and exhaled CO_2 monitoring.

Keywords: infants, newborn, delivery room, neonatal resuscitation, chest compression

1. Introduction

Fortunately, the need for chest compression (CC) or medications in the delivery room is rare. Only about 0.1% of term infants receive these interventions, resulting in approximately 1 million newborn deaths annually worldwide. In addition, chest compression or medications is more frequent in the preterm population (~15%) due to birth asphyxia [1, 2]. Fortunately, the majority of newborn infants successfully make the transition from fetal to neonatal life without any help [3]. An estimated 10% of newborns need help to establish effective ventilation (e.g., positive pressure ventilation, PPV), which remains the most critical step of neonatal resuscitation [3]. However, clinicians struggle to deliver an adequate tidal volume (V_T) [4]. In addition, mask positive pressure ventilation is often impaired by either mask leak or airway obstruction [5]. Manikin studies have further demonstrated that initiation of chest compression increases mask leak and therefore impedes effective ventilation [6, 7]. It is imperative to give optimal ventilation during chest compression to maximize efficacy [8]. Recently, a respiratory function monitor (RFM) has been described to be support the clinical team during simulated [9, 10] and real-time neonatal resuscitation [11–14]. This chapter discusses how an RFM can aid during neonatal resuscitation.

2. Respiratory function monitor

2.1. V_T, gas flow, airway pressure, and exhaled CO_2 monitor

Gas flow, V_T, airway pressure, and *exhaled* CO_2 (ECO_2) can be measured by any respiratory function monitor using a flow sensor placed between a ventilation device and facemask or endotracheal tube [11, 14]. Inspiratory and expiratory tidal volume passing through the sensor can be calculated by any flow sensor (e.g., fixed orifice pneumotach or a hot wire anemometer) by integrating the flow signal [11, 14]. Airway pressure is measured by directly connecting a line to the circuit, which displays peak inflation pressure and positive end expiratory pressure. Any respiratory function monitor continuously displays waves (e.g., pressure, flow, and tidal volume) and numerical values (e.g., airway pressure, tidal volume, and respiratory rate) [11, 14]. In addition, the percentage of mask leak or around a tracheal tube is calculated and displayed. ECO_2 is measured using a non-dispersive infrared absorption technique. According to manufacturers, the accuracy for gas flow is ±0.125 L/min and for ECO_2 is ±2 mmHg.

3. Mask leak

Mask ventilation studies in the delivery room have reported variable mask leak during positive pressure ventilation [4], which can be significantly decreased if mask leak is displayed on an RFM [13]. Using a manikin, Binder-Heschl et al. reported that mask leak significantly increased from 15% during positive pressure ventilation to 32% after chest compression was started [6]. This is further supported by a study by Solevåg et al. who reported that tidal volume delivery is significantly decreased using continuous chest compression with non-synchronized ventilation compared to the current 3:1 cardiopulmonary resuscitation (CPR) [7]. However, when a resuscitation used an RFM to asses mask leak, it was significantly reduced [6]. Unfortunately, the data in newborn infants are sparse and limited to a case report by Li et al. [12]. During chest compression, mask leak was 100% and did not result in an increase in heart rate, suggesting that adequate tidal volume was not delivered (**Figure 1**) [12].

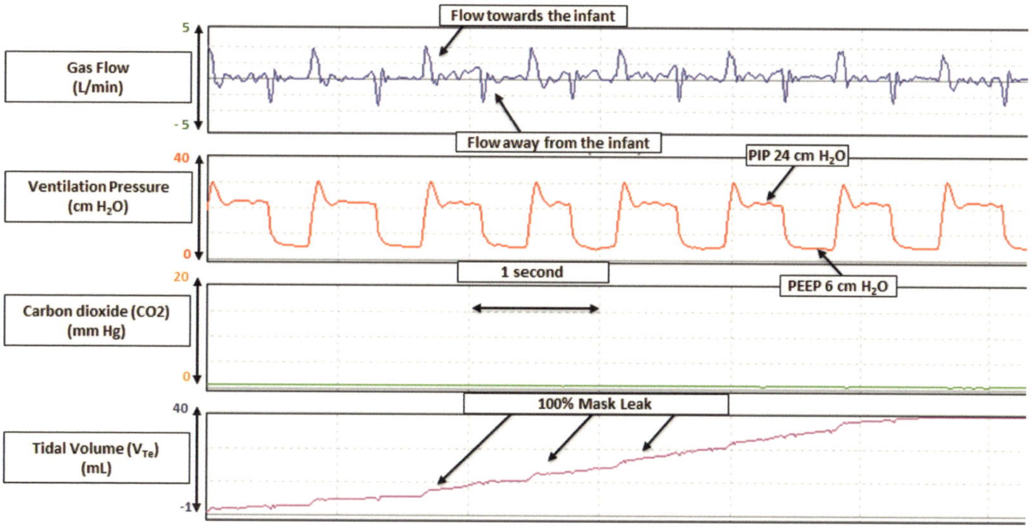

Figure 1. As CC is initiated in an extremely preterm infant, the traces indicate large mask leak. This results in ineffective ventilation and no V_T delivered, which could lead to failure of achieving ROSC.

4. Tidal volume

The purpose of inflations during chest compression is to deliver an adequate tidal volume to facilitate gas exchange [3]. A manikin study reported that tidal volume increases once chest compression was started compared to mask ventilation alone [7]. Interestingly, a further manikin study examined different auditory prompts during simulated neonatal cardiopulmonary resuscitation and reported higher tidal volumes in all groups compared to baseline [15]. These studies suggest a change in tidal volume once chest compressions are initiated. An increase or decrease in tidal volume could cause lung derecruitment, which could hamper oxygenation and therefore return of spontaneous circulation (ROSV) [12]. In a porcine model of neonatal resuscitation, Li et al. recently described that using the current recommendation of 3:1 chest compression to ventilation ratio (**Figure 2**) [3], lung derecruitment occurs [8]. The study further compared continuous chest compressions with asynchronous ventilations and found similar results [8], however, when chest compression superimposed by sustained inflation (CC + SI) (**Figure 3**) [16] improved tidal volume delivery and continuous lung recruitment was observed, potentially leading to better alveolar oxygen delivery and lung aeration.

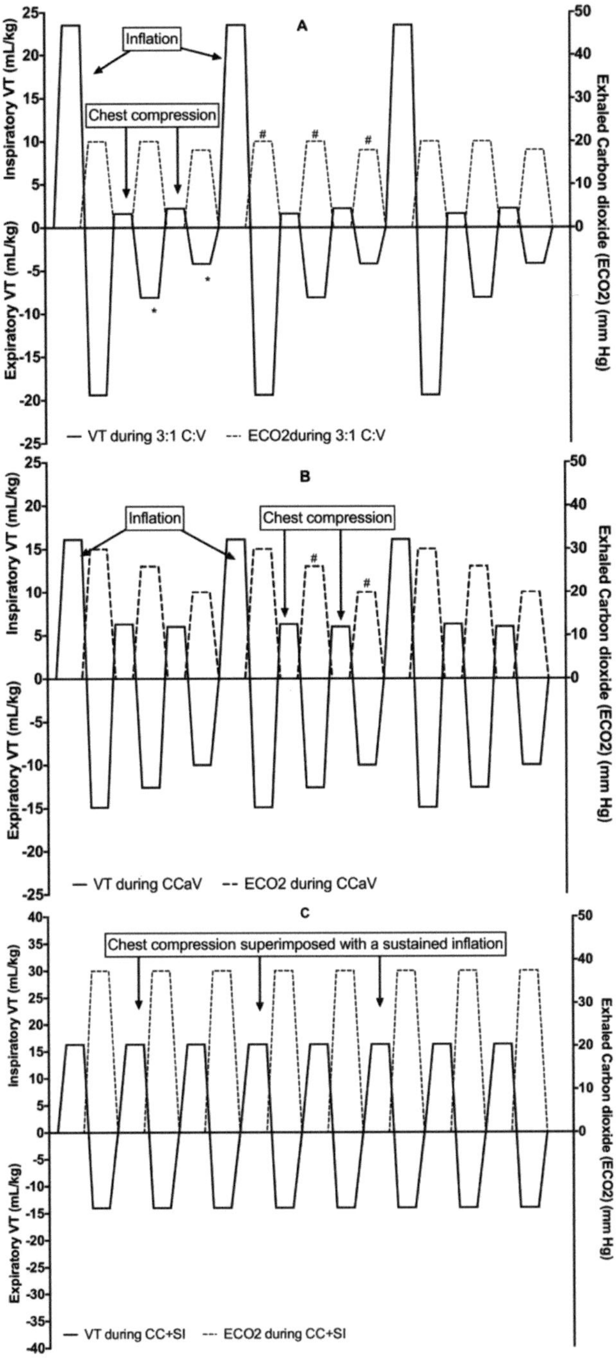

Figure 2. V_T (mL/kg) changes during 3:1 chest compression:ventilation ratio (3:1 C:V) (A), continuous chest compressions and asynchronous ventilations (CCaV) (B), and continuous chest compressions superimposed by sustained inflations (CC + SI) (C). #$p < 0.05$ exhaled CO_2 (ECO_2) compared with CC + SI [8] (with permission).

http://dx.doi.org/10.5772/63510

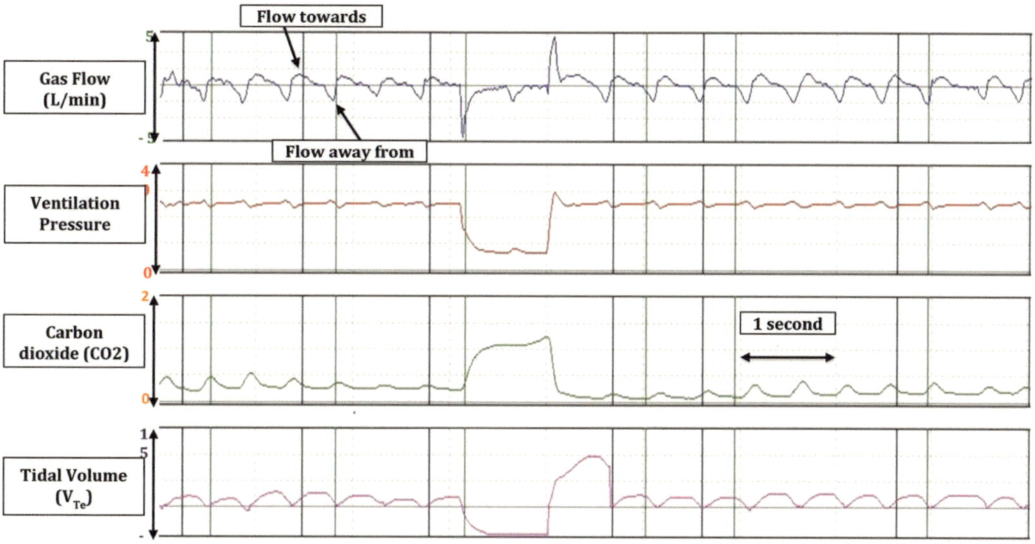

Figure 3. CC superimposed by sustained inflation; adequate lung ventilation and V_T delivery are displayed: (i) adequate gas flow towards and away from the infant; (ii) average V_T of 4 mL/kg is delivered without leak.

5. Exhaled carbon dioxide (ECO_2)

There is increasing evidence that continuous monitoring of exhaled carbon dioxide (ECO_2) can predict rise of heart rate during neonatal transition [17], monitor lung aeration at birth [11, 18–20], and predict return of spontaneous circulation during neonatal cardiopulmonary resuscitation (**Figure 4**) [21]. Blank et al. used a Pedi-Cap during mask positive pressure ventilation and reported a significant increase in heart rate once the Pedi-Cap turned yellow [17]. Similar results have been described in animal models and a further delivery room study [18]. During neonatal cardiopulmonary resuscitation ECO_2 is a reliable parameter to examine return of spontaneous circulation. Chalak et al. reported that an ECO_2 of 14 mmHg was the most reliable indicator for return of spontaneous circulation with 92% sensitivity and 81% specificity [21]. This study suggests that monitoring ECO_2 during cardiopulmonary resuscitation would allow uninterrupted chest compression and potentially could be an indirect indicator of the CC effectiveness. This has been further supported by a recent animal study by Li et al., suggesting that either ECO_2, rate of elimination of CO_2 (VCO_2) or partial pressure of exhaled ($PeCO_2$) could be used to monitor the return of spontaneous circulation [12]. A recent case report of neonatal cardiopulmonary resuscitation in an extremely preterm infant supports this hypothesis where a significant increase in ECO_2 preceded an increase in heart rate and return of spontaneous circulation [12]. ECO_2 monitoring is a non-invasive tool that can be used to predict the return of spontaneous circulation during cardiopulmonary resuscitation.

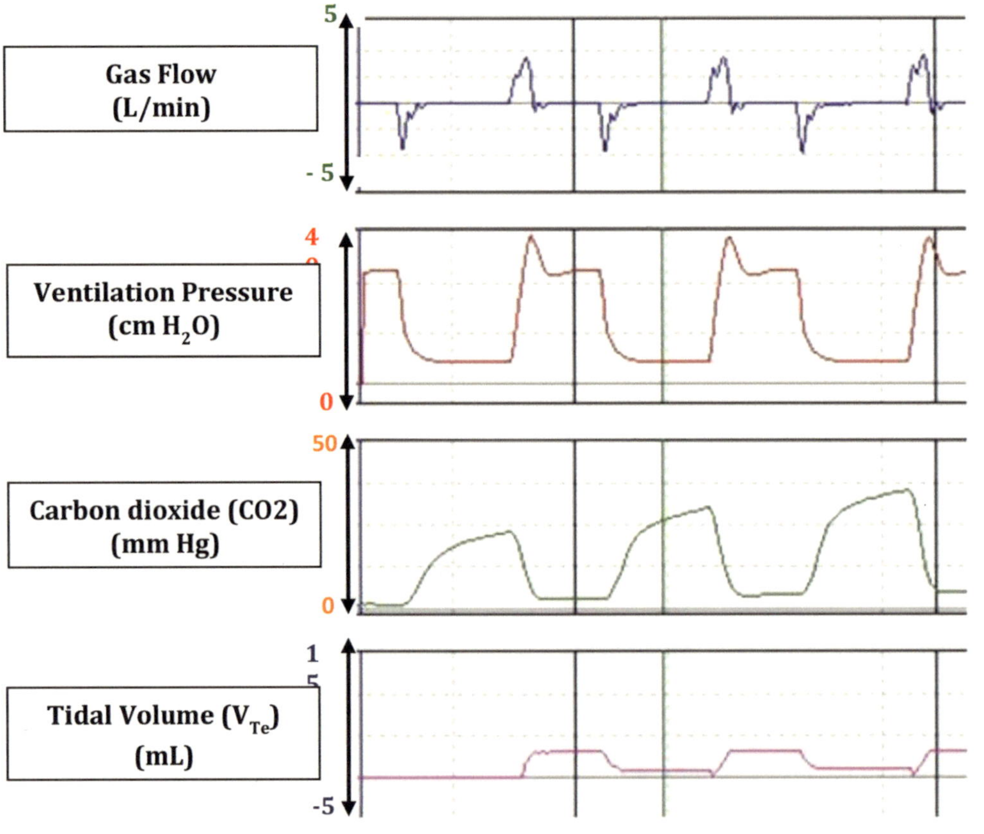

Figure 4. Increasing ECO_2 values suggesting imminent ROSC.

5.1. Partial pressure of exhaled ($PeCO_2$) and rate of elimination of CO_2 (VCO_2)

A recent animal study described VCO_2 and $PECO_2$ values as a clinical indicator during chest compression to achieve the return of spontaneous circulation. VCO_2, or the volume of expired CO_2, reflects changes in both ventilation and perfusion, and therefore ventilation/perfusion (V/Q) matching [22]. Palme-Kilander et al. reported that low VCO_2 values could be due to residual lung fluid, very low tone, or deficient perfusion of the lungs [23]. A recent study in preterm infants reported that higher VCO_2 levels were associated with lung aeration and successful establishment of functional residual capacity [19]. During chest compression, increasing VCO_2 values reflects adequate ventilation, perfusion, and lung aeration [22]. Thus, VCO_2 potentially provides valuable information during neonatal resuscitation.

http://dx.doi.org/10.5772/63510

$PeCO_2$ is a continuous, non-invasive measurement. Since the physiological dead space/tidal volume (V_D/V_T) ratio is never zero, $PeCO_2$ is always lower than the $ETCO_2$ [22]. During resuscitation, there is poor ventilation to perfusion matching, and therefore dead space/tidal volume increases, independent of whether mismatching is either due to impaired perfusion, impaired ventilation, or a mixture of impaired perfusion and ventilation, causing lower $PeCO_2$ [22]. Therefore, $PeCO_2$ is decreased under all conditions of impaired ventilation/perfusion. In the case of ventilation mismatch, $PeCO_2$ is dilute relative to $ETCO_2$, and the $PeCO_2/ETCO_2$ ratio is reduced. In the case of reduced or maldistributed pulmonary blood flow without airway defects, both $PeCO_2$ and $ETCO_2$ would be reduced, resulting in a near normal $PeCO_2/ETCO_2$ ratio. A recent animal study described $PeCO_2$ for the first time in the neonatal population. Newborn piglets who successfully achieved return of spontaneous circulation had significantly higher $PeCO_2$ levels in the latter portion of cardiopulmonary resuscitation, indicating sufficient gas exchange was occurring [22]. Low levels of $PeCO_2$ can only be attributed to poor or low quality of ventilation during cardiopulmonary resuscitation, while decreased levels of both $PeCO_2$ and $ETCO_2$ may signify inadequate pulmonary perfusion due to poor circulation [22]. These findings suggest that monitoring $PeCO_2$ and $ETCO_2$ continuously during cardiopulmonary resuscitation, the clinical team would be able to determine changes in ventilation or perfusion and adjust ventilation to improve either.

6. Conclusion

Using a respiratory function monitor to assess mask leak and tidal volume delivery during neonatal cardiopulmonary resuscitation can help improve mask ventilation. In addition, using exhaled carbon dioxide can predict return of spontaneous circulation during neonatal cardiopulmonary resuscitation.

Abbreviations

CPR cardio pulmonary resuscitation

CC chest compression

CC+SI continuous chest compressions with sustained inflations

ECO_2 exhaled carbon dioxide

PPV positive pressure ventilation

ROSC return of spontaneous circulation

V_T tidal volume

VD/VT physiological dead space/tidal volume

Acknowledgements

MOR is supported by a Molly Towell Perinatal Research Foundation Fellowship. ALS is supported by the Canadian Institute of Health Research (MOP299116) and the South-Eastern Norway Regional Health Authority. GMS is a recipient of the Heart and Stroke Foundation/ University of Alberta Professorship of Neonatal Resuscitation and Heart and Stroke Foundation Canada Research Scholar.

Conflict of Interest: None declared by the authors.

Author details

Georg M Schmölzer[1,2*], Anne Solevåg[1,2], Erica McGinn[1], Megan O'Reilly[1,3] and Po-Yin Cheung[1,2]

*Address all correspondence to: georg.schmoelzer@me.com

1 Centre for the Studies of Asphyxia and Resuscitation, Neonatal Research Unit, Royal Alexandra Hospital, Edmonton, Alberta, Canada

2 Department of Pediatrics, University of Alberta, Edmonton, Alberta, Canada

3 Department of Physiology, University of Alberta, Edmonton, Alberta, Canada

References

[1] Kapadia V, Wyckoff MH. Chest compressions for bradycardia or asystole in neonates. Clin Perinatol 2012;39:833–42.

[2] Wyckoff MH, Perlman J. Cardiopulmonary resuscitation in very low birth weight infants. Pediatrics 2000;106:618–20.

[3] Perlman J, Wyllie JP, Kattwinkel J, Wyckoff MH, Aziz K, Guinsburg R, et al. Part 7: Neonatal resuscitation: 2015 International consensus on cardiopulmonary resuscitation and emergency cardiovascular care science with treatment recommendations. Circulation 2015;132:S204–41.

[4] Schmölzer GM, Kamlin COF, O'Donnell CP, Dawson JA, Morley CJ, Davis PG. Assessment of tidal volume and gas leak during mask ventilation of preterm infants in the delivery room. Arch Dis Child Fetal Neonatal 2010;95:F393–7.

[5] Schmölzer GM, Dawson JA, Kamlin COF, O'Donnell CP, Morley CJ, Davis PG. Airway obstruction and gas leak during mask ventilation of preterm infants in the delivery room. Arch Dis Child Fetal Neonatal 2011;96:F254–7.

[6] Binder-Heschl C, Schmölzer GM, O'Reilly M, Schwaberger B, Pichler G. Human or monitor feedback to improve mask ventilation during simulated neonatal cardiopulmonary resuscitation. Arch Dis Child Fetal Neonatal 2014;99:F120–3.

[7] Solevåg AL, Madland JM, Gjærum E, Nakstad B. Minute ventilation at different compression to ventilation ratios, different ventilation rates, and continuous chest compressions with asynchronous ventilation in a newborn manikin. Scand J Trauma Resusc Emerg Med 2012;20:73.

[8] Li ES-S, Cheung P-Y, O'Reilly M, Schmölzer GM. Change in tidal volume during cardiopulmonary resuscitation in newborn piglets. Arch Dis Child Fetal Neonatal 2015;100:F530–3.

[9] Schilleman K, Witlox RS, Lopriore E, Morley CJ, Walther FJ, te Pas A. Leak and obstruction with mask ventilation during simulated neonatal resuscitation. Arch Dis Child Fetal Neonatal 2010;95:F398–402.

[10] Schmölzer GM, Roehr C. Use of respiratory function monitors during simulated neonatal resuscitation. Klin Padiatr 2011;223:261–6.

[11] van Os S, Cheung P-Y, Pichler G, Aziz K, O'Reilly M, Schmölzer GM. Exhaled carbon dioxide can be used to guide respiratory support in the delivery room. Acta Paediatr 2014;103:796–806.

[12] Li ES-S, Cheung P-Y, Pichler G, Aziz K, Schmölzer GM. Respiratory function and near infrared spectroscopy recording during cardiopulmonary resuscitation in an extremely preterm newborn. Neonatology 2014;105:200–4.

[13] Schmölzer GM, Morley CJ, Wong C, Dawson JA, Kamlin COF, Donath S, et al. Respiratory function monitor guidance of mask ventilation in the delivery room: a feasibility study. J Pediatr 2012;160:377–381.e2.

[14] Schmölzer GM, Kamlin COF, Dawson JA, te Pas A, Morley CJ, Davis PG. Respiratory monitoring of neonatal resuscitation. Arch Dis Child Fetal Neonatal 2010;95:F295–303.

[15] Roehr C, Schmölzer GM, Thio M, Dawson JA, Dold SK, Schmalisch G, et al. How ABBA may help improve neonatal resuscitation training: auditory prompts to enable coordination of manual inflations and chest compressions. J Paediatr Child Health 2014;50:444–8.

[16] Schmölzer GM, O'Reilly M, LaBossiere J, Lee T-F, Cowan S, Qin S, et al. Cardiopulmonary resuscitation with chest compressions during sustained inflations: a new technique of neonatal resuscitation that improves recovery and survival in a neonatal porcine model. Circulation 2013;128:2495–503.

[17] Blank D, Rich W, Leone TA, Garey D, Finer N. Pedi-cap color change precedes a significant increase in heart rate during neonatal resuscitation. Resuscitation 2014;85:1568–72.

[18] Hooper SB, Fouras A, Siew M, Wallace MJ, Kitchen M, te Pas A, et al. Expired CO_2 levels indicate degree of lung aeration at birth. PLoS One 2013;8:e70895.

[19] Kang LJ, Cheung P-Y, Pichler G, O'Reilly M, Aziz K, Schmölzer GM. Monitoring lung aeration during respiratory support in preterm infants at birth. PLoS One 2014;9:e102729.

[20] Kong JY, Rich W, Finer N, Leone TA. Quantitative end-tidal carbon dioxide monitoring in the delivery room: a randomized controlled trial. J Pediatr 2013;163:104–8.e1.

[21] Chalak LF, Barber CA, Hynan L, Garcia D, Christie L, Wyckoff MH. End-tidal CO_2 detection of an audible heart rate during neonatal cardiopulmonary resuscitation after asystole in asphyxiated piglets. Pediatr Res 2011;69:401–5.

[22] Li ES-S, Cheung P-Y, O'Reilly M, LaBossiere J, Lee T-F, Cowan S, et al. Exhaled CO_2 parameters as a tool to assess ventilation-perfusion mismatching during neonatal resuscitation in a swine model of neonatal asphyxia. PLoS One 2016;11:e0146524–11.

[23] Palme-Kilander C, Tunell R, Chiwei Y. Pulmonary gas exchange immediately after birth in spontaneously breathing infants. Arch Dis Child 1993;68:6–10.

Chapter 2

Alternative Therapies for the Management of Respiratory Distress Syndrome

Alejandro González-Garay and
Vicente González-Bustamante

Additional information is available at the end of the chapter

http://dx.doi.org/10.5772/63384

Abstract

Respiratory distress syndrome (RDS) is a disorder caused by a deficiency of surface-active agent called pulmonary surfactant, in the pulmonary alveoli. This deficiency leads the alveoli to collapse, impeding air entry, gas exchange, and oxygenation in newborns. Conventional treatment involves exogenous surfactant administration, ventilation, and hydroelectrolytic management.

However, there are alternative treatments to prevent RDS that can be administered to pregnant women (steroids, thyrotropin-releasing hormone, and ambroxol) or to newborns in their first few hours of life (continuous positive airway pressure, prophylactic surfactant in single or multiple doses, and digoxin). These approaches may be effective and cost less than conventional treatment. Conventional treatment requires trained medical personnel to attend to the newborn, ventilation, temperature control, and electrolytic and nutritional support, which can cost up to USD 14,226 per event.

This chapter seeks to analyze the effectiveness of each of these alternative treatments in preventing RDS in preterm newborns, so that it can be applied in communities with limited resources.

Keywords: ambroxol, respiratory distress syndrome, antenatal steroids, preterm birth, alternative therapies

1. Introduction

The lungs are composed of different structures. The alveoli are the functional units of the lungs that allow oxygen gas (O_2) from the environment to be exchanged for carbon dioxide (CO_2) from the bloodstream.

In order for this process to take place, contact between the air-filled alveoli and the capillaries of the lung is essential. However, certain conditions can affect this process by preventing air from entering the alveoli, diminishing blood flow in pulmonary capillaries, or impeding alveolus-capillary contact, which hampers gas exchange and leads to decreased O_2 and increased CO_2 levels in the blood [1].

Alveoli comprise (a) type I pneumocytes, cells that provide shape and support and (b) type II pneumocytes, cells responsible for producing the surface-active agent called pulmonary surfactant. A surfactant is a substance made up of phospholipids (80%), proteins (12%), and neutral lipids (8%). Surfactants decrease the surface tension inside the alveoli. When there is insufficient surfactant, the alveoli collapse, preventing air entry and gas exchange. This is accompanied by a decrease in O_2 in the tissues and a gradual increase in respiratory effort, leading to this disorder being known as respiratory distress syndrome (RDS) [1–3].

This disorder affects up to 30% of premature newborns (<37 weeks of gestation) and accounts for 9.3–12% of hospital admissions to neonatal intensive care units [4–6]. Some studies have reported that the following factors are linked to the development of RDS: birth by cesarean section, gestational diabetes, meconium aspiration, and neonatal asphyxia [7].

Conventional treatment, which has been shown to reduce mortality rates by up to 18%, involves the exogenous administration of natural or synthetic surfactant at a dose of 100 mg/kg, up to 2–3 times, once RDS is diagnosed. The treatment also involves the use of mechanical ventilation, temperature control in an incubator, and electrolytic and nutritional support. However, this treatment has multiple adverse effects, such as pneumothorax, bronchopulmonary dysplasia, and retinopathy secondary to ventilation support and the continuous administration of supplemental oxygen over prolonged periods, malnutrition, and infections [2, 8].

As a consequence, many researchers have studied alternatives to prevent the development of RDS and reduce the frequency of these complications.

2. Alternative treatments for the prevention of RDS

The following are some treatments designed to prevent the development of RDS in newborns.

2.1. Early administration of surfactant

Numerous studies have reported that the administration of surfactant in the first few hours of life prior to the development of RDS reduces the mortality rate of preterm newborns. In 2012,

http://dx.doi.org/10.5772/63384

Bahadue and Soll carried out a systematic review of six clinical trials involving 3577 preterm newborns and analyzed the effectiveness of administering surfactant in the first 2 hours of life. The authors found a significant reduction in the risk of death [RR 0.84 (0.74–0.95)] compared to delayed selective surfactant administration with neonates with established RDS [9] (**Figure 1**).

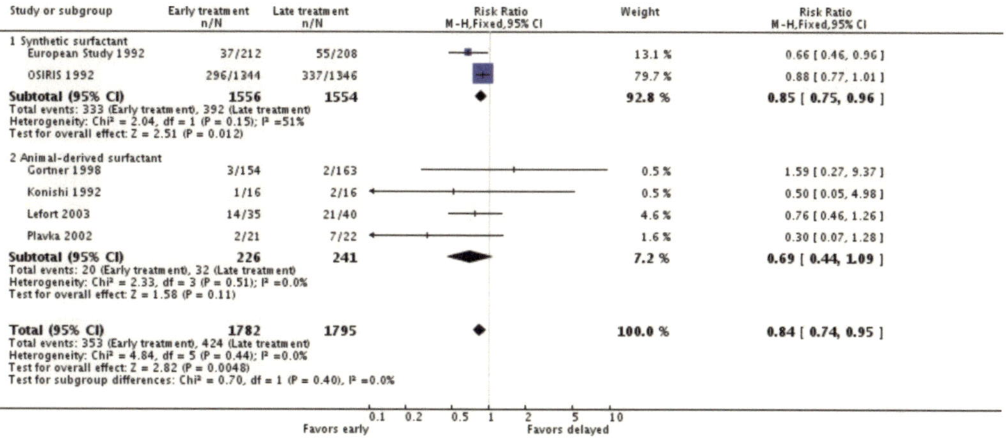

Figure 1. Early vs delayed administration of surfactant (risk of death).

Bahadue also analyzed adverse effects in patients that received early administration of surfactant and reported that there was a decrease in the risk of developing chronic lung disease [RR 0.69 (0.55–0.86)], pneumothorax [RR 0.69 (0.59–0.82)], pulmonary interstitial emphysema [RR 0.60 (0.41–0.89)], and bronchopulmonary dysplasia [RR 0.94 (0.88–1.00)] [9] (**Figures 2–5**).

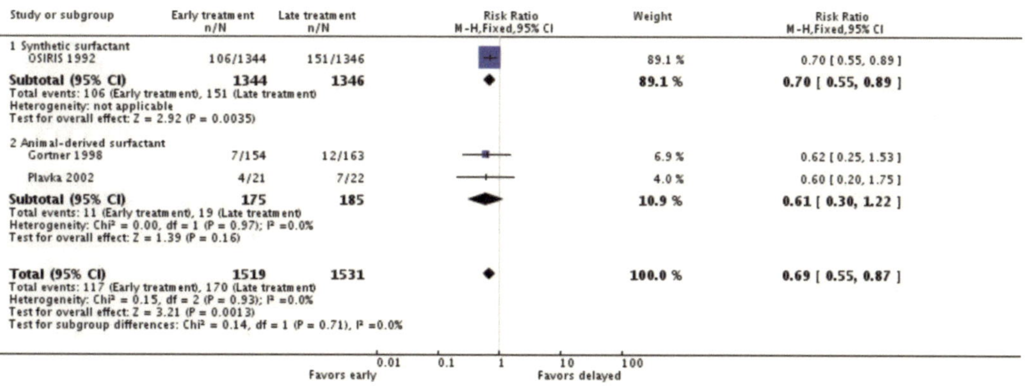

Figure 2. Early vs delayed selective surfactant treatment (chronic lung disease).

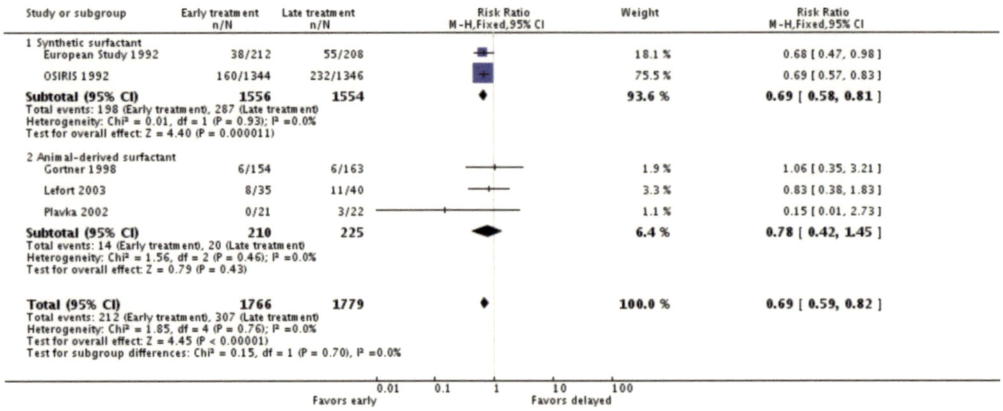

Figure 3. Early vs delayed selective surfactant treatment (pneumothorax).

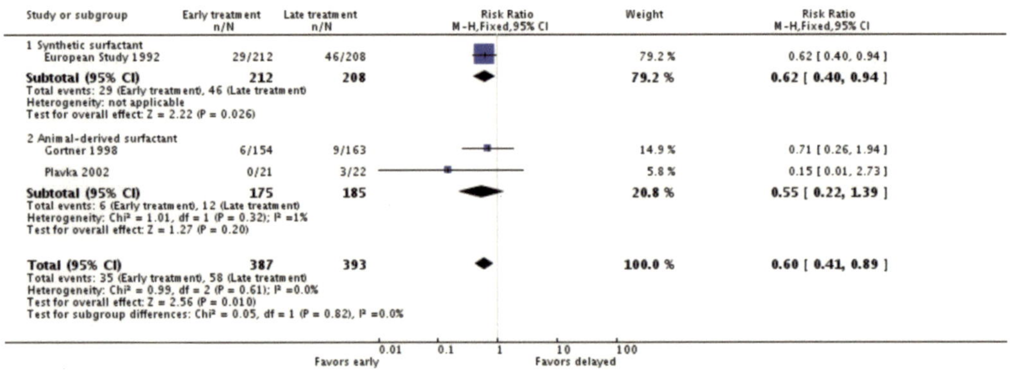

Figure 4. Early vs delayed selective surfactant treatment (pulmonary interstitial emphysema).

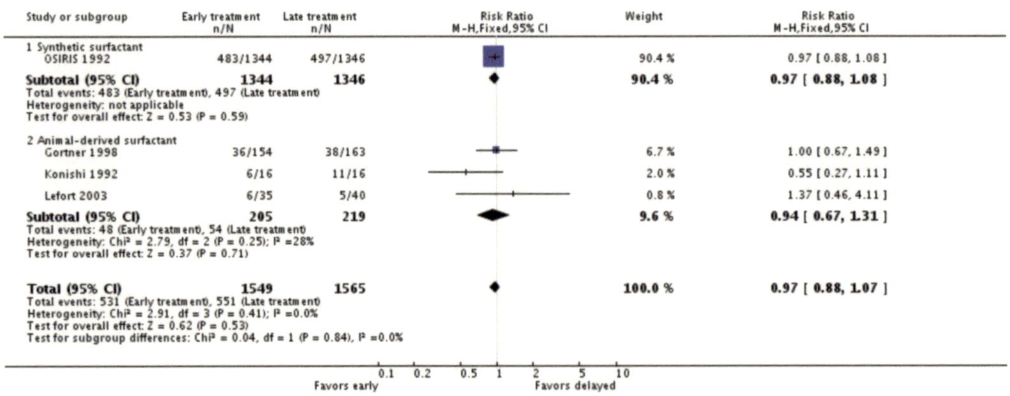

Figure 5. Early vs delayed selective surfactant treatment (bronchopulmonary dysplasia).

http://dx.doi.org/10.5772/63384

2.2. Administration of multiple doses of surfactant

Some researchers have carried out clinical trials to determine the effectiveness of administering multiple doses of surfactant to newborns to prevent RDS or reduce its complications. In 2009, Soll and Ozek carried out a systematic review to investigate whether this alternative treatment could decrease the risk of RDS and complications in preterm newborns. Only three clinical trials could be included in the review, but the authors concluded from these that there was a decrease in the risk of developing pneumothorax for neonates that received up to a maximum of four doses of surfactant spaced 6–12 hours apart compared to those who received single doses [RR 0.51 (0.30–0.88)]. There was a non-significant decrease in the risk of death for newborns who received multiple doses of surfactant [RR 0.63 (0.39–1.02)]. They concluded that the ability to give multiple doses of surfactant to infants with ongoing respiratory insufficiency leads to improved clinical outcome and appears to be the most effective treatment policy (**Figures 6** and 7) [10].

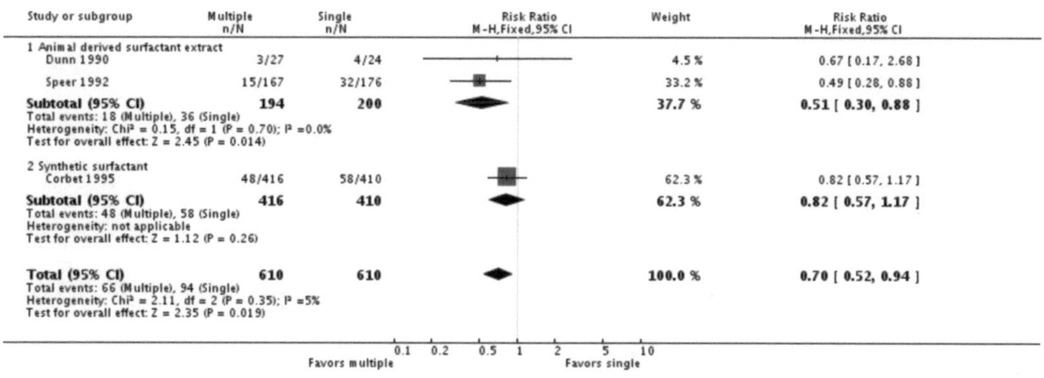

Figure 6. Multiple vs single doses of pulmonary treatment (pneumothorax).

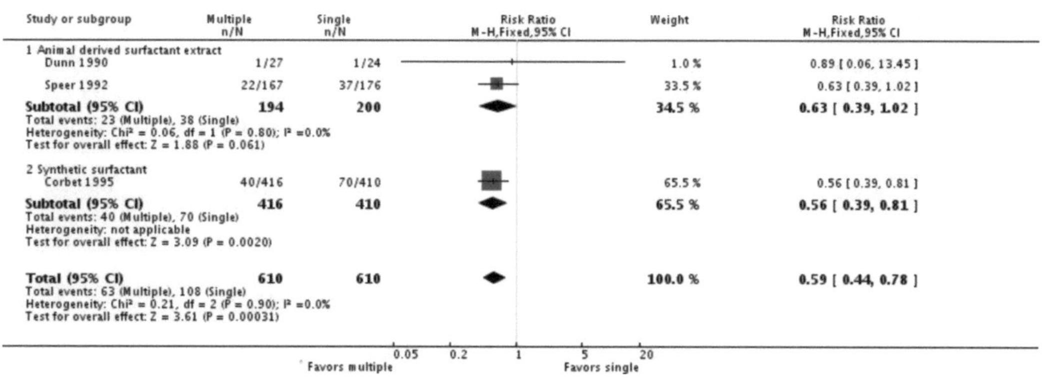

Figure 7. Multiple vs single doses of pulmonary surfactant (mortality).

2.3. Early application of continuous positive airway pressure (CPAP)

CPAP is an alternative treatment for newborns with RDS that involves the application of a type of respiratory support that applies air at low pressure in a continuous manner to keep the airway open. This treatment increases functional residual capacity and oxygenation with fewer secondary effects [11].

It has been observed that this type of respiratory support carries a lower risk of secondary complications such as barotrauma, pneumothorax, and pulmonary emphysema, among others. Recent studies of CPAP application in premature neonates in the first few minutes of life have shown that the risk of death is lower [RR 0.68 (0.5–1.92)] than for neonates who receive conventional ventilation. It has also been reported that the early application of CPAP in patients who developed RDS and received conventional treatment reduced the duration of mechanical ventilation (25 vs. 28 days) [12].

These findings were confirmed in a systematic review by Bahadue, who reported that the early application of CPAP and the selective administration of surfactants in preterm neonates reduced the risk of death compared to newborns who received only prophylactic surfactant [RR 0.84 (0.74–0.95)] [9].

To study long-term outcomes, Vaucher and colleagues carried out a follow-up assessment at 22 months of 1310 neonates that had been treated with CPAP to prevent RDS and found a decrease in the frequency of neurological and respiratory problems compared to patients treated with conventional therapy involving mechanical ventilation [RR 0.93 (0.78–1.10)] [13], similar findings were observed in the prospective study performed by Stevens and colleagues in 918 infants; those who received CPAP had fewer episodes of wheezing, respiratory illnesses, and visits to emergency room for breathing problems compared to infants who received conventional therapy [28.9% vs. 36.5%, 47.7% vs. 55.2%, and 68% vs. 72.9% ($p < 0.05$), respectively] [14].

On the basis of these results, the American Academy of Pediatrics recommends the early use of CPAP in conjunction with surfactant administration as an alternative to prevent RDS in preterm newborns [15].

2.4. Administration of digoxin

In 1955, Lendrum suggested that cardiac insufficiency secondary to pulmonary edema was a predisposing factor for RDS. Several clinical trials were carried out to determine whether the administration of digoxin in the first few hours of life would improve heart contractility and reduce the risk of developing RDS [16, 17].

As part of a systematic review in 2011, Soll and Ozek analyzed the efficacy of digoxin application in preventing RDS at doses of 0.01–0.06 mg/kg every 12 hours in 212 preterm newborns. They found that, despite improvements to cardiac insufficiency, there was no significant reduction in mortality compared to newborns who did not receive digoxin [RR 1.27 (0.78–2.07)]. The authors concluded that although hemodynamic disturbances play a role in the overall pathogenesis of RDS, the specific contribution of early congestive heart failure does

http://dx.doi.org/10.5772/63384

not appear to be significant factor in RDS, and the treatment with digoxin has no proven value in infants solely affected with RDS [18] (**Figure 8**).

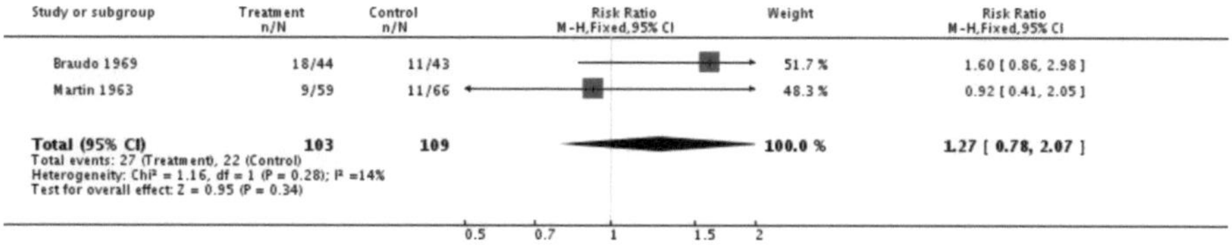

Figure 8. Digoxin vs placebo for preventing or treating respiratory distress syndrome (mortality).

2.5. Administration of thyrotropin-releasing hormone and antenatal steroids

In 1972, Liggins and Howie demonstrated that the administration of steroids (betamethasone) to pregnant women at risk of giving birth prematurely reduced the risk of their newborns developing RDS [RR 0.69 (0.59–0.73)] because the steroid passes through the placenta, reaches the fetal pulmonary alveoli, and stimulates the production of surfactant by type II pneumocytes. However, the use of this treatment did not become commonplace until 1987. It has since reduced the rate of neonatal mortality and is the preventive therapy of choice for obstetricians [19, 20].

Later, Liggins found that the administration of thyrotropin-releasing hormone (TRH) in combination with antenatal steroids increased the production of phospholipids and the distension of fetal sheep' lungs [19]. In 2013, Crowther carried out a systematic review analyzing 4600 pregnant women who were administered TRH and steroids prior to delivery. However, no significant differences were observed in terms of reducing the risk of death for premature newborns [RR 1.05 (0.86–1.27)] (**Figure 9**) or prevention of RDS compared to neonates born to women who received antenatal betamethasone therapy [RR 1.05 (0.91–1.22)] (**Figure 10**). However, it was observed that the administration of the combination of TRH and antenatal steroids did significantly increase the risk of adverse effects such as nausea, vomiting, and headaches [RR 3.92 (3.13–4.92), RR 2.35 (1.35–4.09), and RR 1.73 (1.36–2.22), respectively] (**Figures 11–13**) [21].

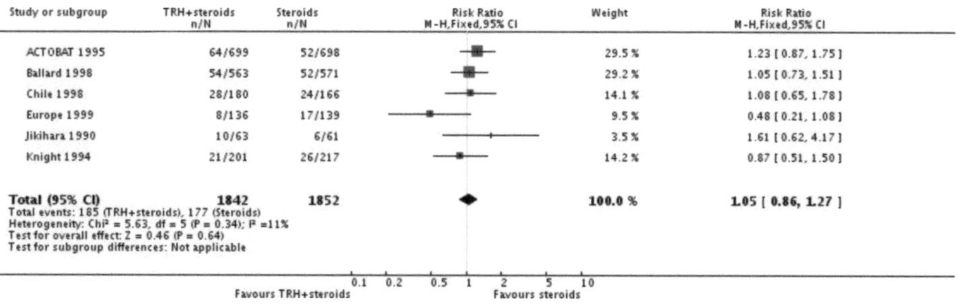

Figure 9. Thyrotropin-releasing hormone + steroids vs steroids alone for RDS (mortality).

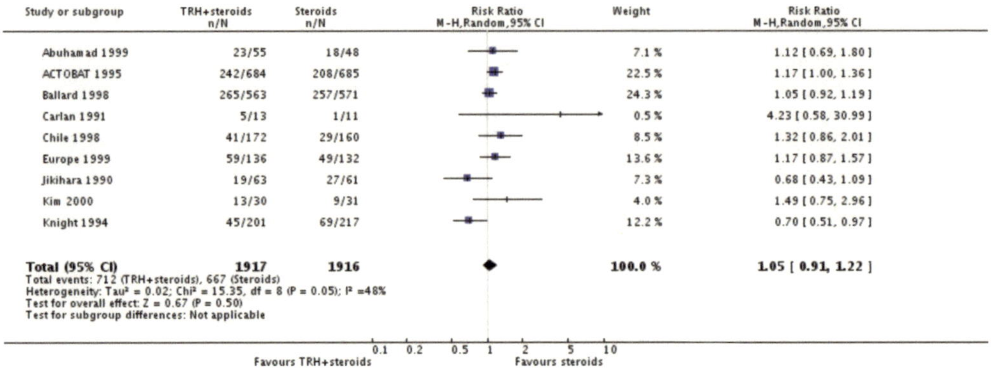

Figure 10. Thyrotropin-releasing hormone + steroids vs steroids alone for respiratory distress syndrome.

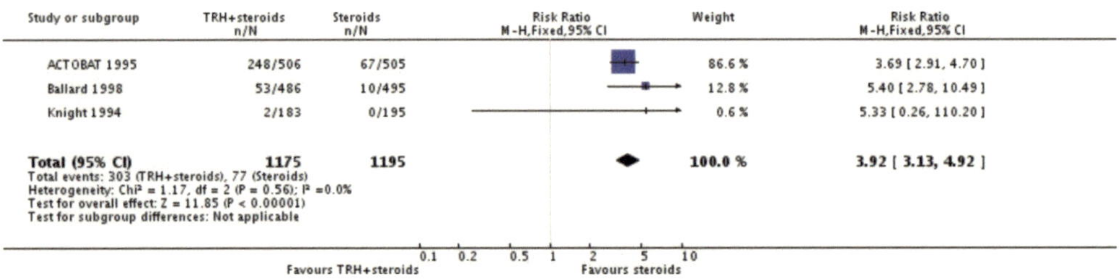

Figure 11. Thyrotropin-releasing hormone + steroids vs steroids alone for RDS (nausea).

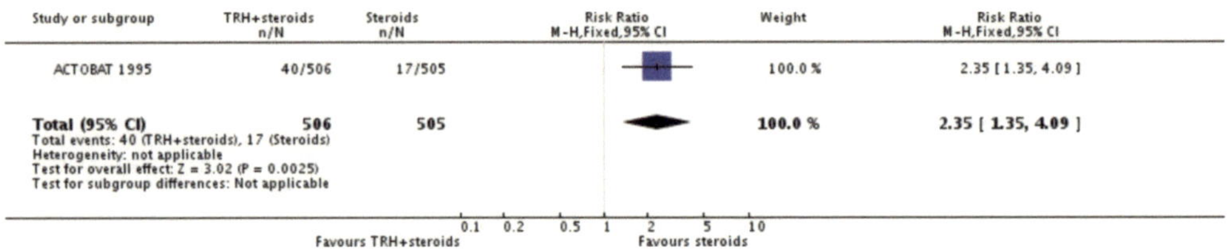

Figure 12. Thyrotropin-releasing hormone + steroids vs steroids alone for RDS (vomiting).

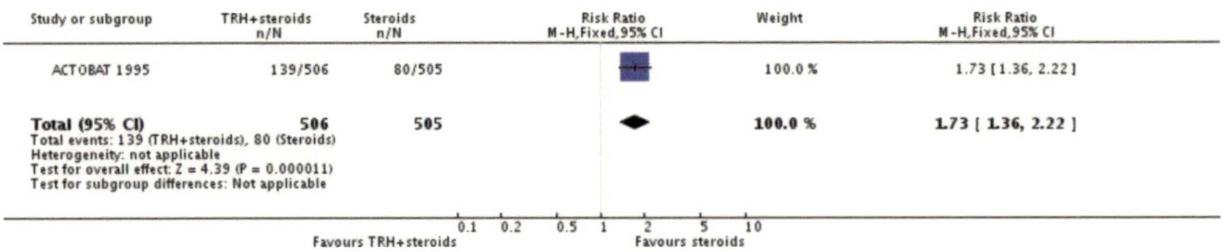

Figure 13. Thyrotropin-releasing hormone + steroids vs steroids alone for RDS (headaches).

http://dx.doi.org/10.5772/63384

2.6. Administration of magnesium sulfate

The administration of magnesium sulfate to pregnant women is used by obstetricians to inhibit labor and birth before 37 weeks of gestation by altering the union and distribution of calcium in the muscle fibers of the uterus, thus reducing the frequency of contractions [22].

In 2015, McNamara carried out a systematic review to analyze the efficacy and safety of magnesium sulfate (4 g loading dose and 2–5 g/h via infusion) administered to 360 pregnant women at less than 37 weeks of gestation to inhibit preterm labor. McNamara observed that this treatment reduces the risk of developing RDS [RR 0.31 (0.11–0.88)] and decreases the time that neonates spend in intensive care [MD −3.10 (0–5.48 to −0.72 days)]. However, there is too little evidence available to recommend the regular use of this treatment (**Figures 14** and **15**) [23].

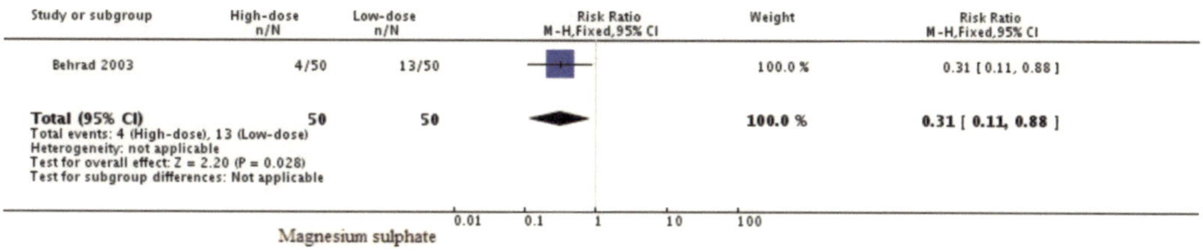

Figure 14. Magnesium sulfate for respiratory distress syndrome.

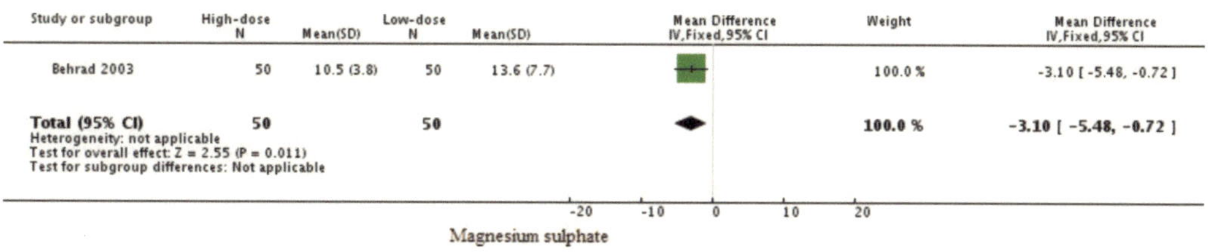

Figure 15. Magnesium sulfate for RDS (days of stay neonatal intensive care unit).

2.7. Administration of ambroxol

Ambroxol is a metabolite derived from bromhexine that increases the movement of cilia in the cells of the respiratory tract, facilitating the transport of mucus in the airway and inhibiting the activity of lysosomal phospholipase, the enzyme responsible for the degradation of pulmonary surfactant [24].

Laoag-Fernandez and Seifart carried out several clinical studies to analyze the effectiveness of ambroxol as an alternative treatment in the prevention of RDS because it allows easily reaching the fetus through placental circulation. These studies allowed Gonzalez to carry out a systematic review in 2014 [25].

The systematic review included 14 clinical trials analyzing 1047 pregnant women at risk of preterm birth who were administered a daily 1 g dose of ambroxol for a week.

The results of the review showed a reduction in the risk of neonates developing RDS compared to treatments in which women were administered antenatal steroids (betamethasone) or a placebo [RR 0.79 (0.59–1.07) and RR 0.74 (0.46–1.20), respectively] (**Figures 16** and **17**) [25].

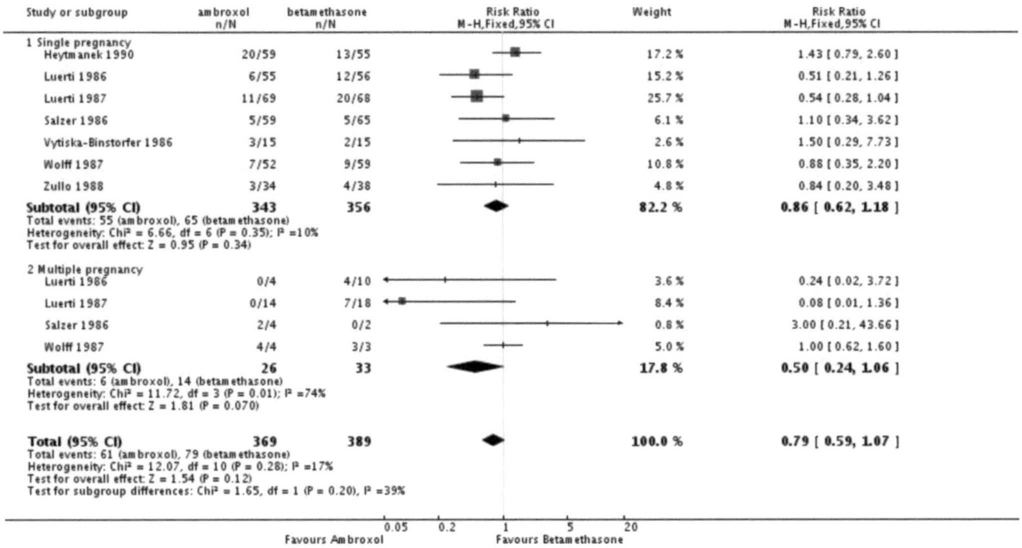

Figure 16. Ambroxol vs betamethasone for respiratory distress syndrome.

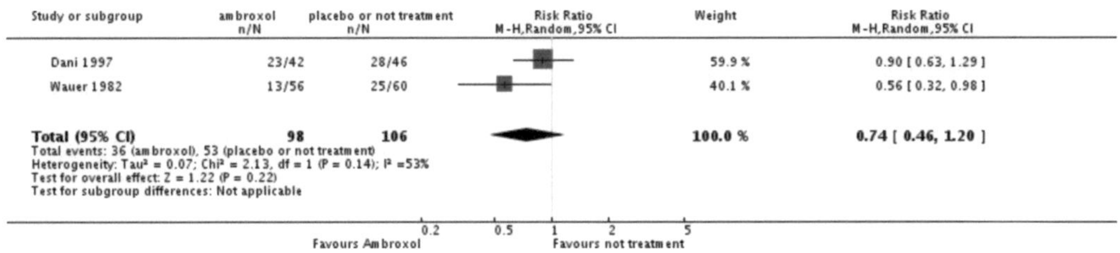

Figure 17. Ambroxol vs placebo or no treatment for respiratory distress syndrome.

3. Conclusions

We can see that although there are multiple alternative treatment options to prevent preterm newborns from developing RDS, their effectiveness has not yet been proven (with the exception of prenatal steroid administration) with evidence that is strong enough due to a lack of studies with larger numbers of participants and sound methodology. Nevertheless, it is possible that these might be viable treatments in communities that do not have the financial resources or the medical care required to attend to these patients. Conventional treatments require trained medical personnel who can attend deliveries and care for premature neonates in hospital units that have the necessary infrastructure as well as mechanical ventilators, temperature control systems, antibiotics for infection control, and intravenous solutions to maintain nutritional and hydroelectrolytic homeostasis.

In 2014, Martínez-Valverde and colleagues carried out a study to estimate the costs of providing care to newborns with RDS in public hospitals in Mexico and found that, on average, the cost per patient per event can reach USD 14,226, without accounting for the cost of treating secondary conditions [26].

Undoubtedly, more studies need to be carried out to strengthen the evidence supporting the use of these alternative treatments. However, they could be a sustainable option in communities with limited financial resources because they are more readily available and have fewer adverse effects and lower costs than conventional treatment.

Author details

Alejandro González-Garay[1*] and Vicente González-Bustamante[2]

*Address all correspondence to: pegasso.100@hotmail.com

1 Methodology Research Unit, National Institute of Pediatrics, Mexico City, Mexico

2 Autonomous Metropolitan University, Mexico City, Mexico

References

[1] Sánchez C, Torres J. Pulmonary Surfactant. Rev. Ped. Elec. 2004;1(1):45–50. ISSN: 0718–0918.

[2] Soll R. Synthetic surfactant for respiratory distress syndrome in preterm infants. Cochrane Database of Systematic Reviews 1998;(3): CD001149. DOI: 10.1002/14651858.CD001149.

[3] Stark AR, Frantz ID. Respiratory distress syndrome. Pediatric Clinics of North America 1986;33(3):533–544.

[4] Kumar A, Bhat BV. Epidemiology of respiratory distress of newborns. Indian J Pediatr. 1996;63(1):93–8.

[5] Sarasqueta P de, Basso G, Pataro MC, Colombrero E, Rodríguez H, González J, et al. Estudio epidemiológico del síndrome de dificultad respiratoria en el recién nacido. AACN Clinical Issues in Critical Care Nursing 1986;28(119):70–7.

[6] Roberts D, Dalziel S. Antenatal corticosteroids for accelerating fetal lung maturation for women at risk of preterm birth. CochraneDatabase of Systematic Reviews 2006; (3):CD004454.

[7] Hansen T, Corbet A. Disorders of the transition. In: Taeush W, Ballard R editor(s). Avery's Diseases of the Newborn. 7a. Mexico: Harcourt, 2000: 602–13.

[8] Udaeta E, Alfaro M. Respiratory Distress Syndrome in the newborn. Neonatology Clínic. Mexico: McGraw Hill, 2004:250–80. ISBN: 9701041216.

[9] Bahadue FL, Soll R. Early versus delayed selective surfactant treatment for neonatal respiratory distress syndrome. Cochrane Database of Systematic Reviews 2012, Issue 11. Art. No.: CD001456. DOI: 10.1002/14651858.CD001456.pub2.

[10] Soll R, Özek E. Multiple versus single doses of exogenous surfactant for the prevention or treatment of neonatal respiratory distress syndrome. Cochrane Database of Systematic Reviews 2009;(1):CD000141. DOI: 10.1002/14651858.CD000141.pub2

[11] Piñeros J, Correa M, Andrade M, Roa M. Neonatal Respiratory Distress by deficit of surfactant. In: Ucrós S, Mejía N editors. Pediatrics practice evidence-based guides 2a. Ed. Colombia: Editorial Médica Panamericana, 2009:62–5. ISBN: 978–9588443–02–7.

[12] Morley C, Davis P, Doyle L, Brion L, Hascoet J, Carlin J; COIN Trial Investigators. Nasal CPAP or intubation at birth for very preterm infants. New England Journal of Medicine 2008;358(7):700–708. DOI: 10.1056/NEJMoa072788

[13] Vaucher Y, Peralta-Carcelen M, Finer NN; SUPPORT Study Group of the Eunice Kennedy Shriver NICHD Neonatal Research Network. Neurodevelopmental outcomes in the early CPAP and pulse oximetry trial. New England Journal of Medicine 2012;367(26):2495–2504. DOI: 10.1056/NEJMoa1208506

[14] Stevens T, Finer N, Carlo W, Szilagyi P, Phelps D, Walsh M, et al. Respiratory outcomes of the surfactant positive pressure and oximetry randomized trial (SUPPORT). Journal of Pediatrics 2014;165(2):240–249.e4. DOI: 10.1016/j.jpeds.2014.02.054

[15] Committe on Fetus and Newborn; American Academy of Pediatrics. Respiratory support in preterm infants at birth. Pediatrics 2014;13381:171–174. DOI: 10.1542/peds. 2013-3442

[16] Lendrum FC. The 'pulmonary hyaline membrane' as a manifestation of heart failure in the newborn infant. Journal of Pediatrics 1955;47:149–156. DOI: 10.1016/S0022-3476(55)80025-X

[17] Stahlman MT. Adaptation to Extra-Uterine Life. Report of 31st Ross Conference on Pediatric Research. Columbus, OH: Ross Laboratories, 1959. Class Number: WS 420 R823A 1958.

[18] Soll R, Özek E. Digoxin for preventing or treating neonatal respiratory distress syndrome. Cochrane Database of Systematic Reviews 2011, Issue 1. Art. No.: CD001080. DOI: 10.1002/14651858.CD001080.pub2

[19] Liggins GC, Schellenberg JC. Synergism of cortisol and thyrotropin-releasing hormone in lung maturation in fetal sheep. Journal of Applied Physiology 1988;65(4):1880–1884. ISSN: 1522–1601

[20] Roberts D, Dalziel SR. Antenatal corticosteroids for accelerating fetal lung maturation for women at risk of preterm birth. Cochrane Database of Systematic Reviews 2006, (3): CD004454. DOI: HYPERLINK "http://dx.doi.org/10.1002/14651858.CD004454.pub2"10.1002/14651858.CD004454.pub2.

[21] Crowther CA, Alfirevic Z, Han S, Haslam RR. Thyrotropin-releasing hormone added to corticosteroids for women at risk of preterm birth for preventing neonatal respiratory disease. Cochrane Database of Systematic Reviews 2013, Issue 11. Art. No.: CD000019. DOI: 10.1002/14651858.CD000019.pub3.

[22] Lewis DF. Magnesium sulfate: the first-line tocolytic. Obstetrics and Gynecology Clinics of North America 2005;32(3):485–500. DOI: 10.1016/j.ogc.2005.03.002

[23] McNamara HC, Crowther CA, Brown J. Different treatment regimens of magnesium sulphate for tocolysis in women in preterm labour. Cochrane Database of Systematic Reviews 2015, Issue 12. Art. No.: CD011200. DOI: 10.1002/14651858.CD011200.pub2.

[24] Disse BG. The pharmacology of ambroxol—review and new results. European Journal of Respiratory Diseases 1987;153:255–262.

[25] Gonzalez Garay AG, Reveiz L, Velasco Hidalgo L, Solis Galicia C. Ambroxol for women at risk of preterm birth for preventing neonatal respiratory distress syndrome. Cochrane Database of Systematic Reviews 2014, Issue 10. Art. No.: CD009708. DOI: 10.1002/14651858.CD009708.pub2.

[26] Martínez-Valderde S, Castro-Ríos A, Salinas-Escudero G, Villasis-Keever M, Garduño-Espinosa J, Muñoz-Hernández O. Direct medical costs of neonatal respiratory distress syndrome in two specialized public hospitals in Mexico. Salud Pública de México 2014;56(6):612–618. ISSN: 0036–3634

Chapter 3

Respiratory Management of the Newborn with an Omphalocele

Joanne Baerg, Arul Thirumoorthi and
Andrew Hopper

Additional information is available at the end of the chapter

http://dx.doi.org/10.5772/63735

Abstract

Despite advances in neonatal care, infants with omphalocele have a mortality rate ranging between 5% and 25%. Respiratory insufficiency is a common clinical challenge and an independent predictor of mortality in these infants. The causes of respiratory failure are diverse and are not well understood. This chapter discusses the unique aspects of respiratory management in omphalocele infants. The authors have chosen references in this chapter with appropriate sample size, variable comparisons, regression analyses, and documented median follow-up times. Omphalocele is rare; therefore, the case reports of chapter references have important information.

Omphalocele infants are sometimes born with inadequate lung volume to support survival. Prenatal predictors of pulmonary hypoplasia are discussed in the context of fetal magnetic resonance imaging (MRI) and postnatal clinical-radiologic correlation studies. Two recent retrospective articles explain the unique aspects of pulmonary hypertension in omphalocele infants and distinguish it from pulmonary hypoplasia. The avoidance of abdominal compartment syndrome at the time of omphalocele closure is discussed. Clinical strategies that improve the respiratory care of these infants, based on Specific definitions and diagnoses, may reduce the high mortality rate.

Keywords: respiratory insufficiency, pulmonary hypoplasia, pulmonary hypertension, abdominal compartment syndrome, extracorporeal membrane oxygenator, delayed repair

1. Introduction

Omphalocele is a congenital ventral defect of the umbilical ring with herniation of the abdominal viscera. The reported incidence is 1 in 6000 live births [1]. If omphalocele is diagnosed in the first trimester, over 30% of fetuses die in utero [2, 3]. Despite advances in neonatal care, for live-born infants, the mortality rate remains between 5% and 25% [4].

Postnatal management includes protection of the herniated viscera, prevention of hypothermia, gastric decompression, and maintenance of cardiopulmonary stability [5].

Respiratory insufficiency at birth is reported as an independent predictor of mortality for infants with omphalocele, but the causes are diverse [1]. Respiratory insufficiency in neonates is generally defined as hypoxemia in room air with progressive respiratory and metabolic acidosis and the need for mechanical ventilation within 24 hours of birth [1].

In this chapter, giant and nongiant omphaloceles are compared, as giant omphalocele infants have a more complex postnatal course and more respiratory difficulties.

Prenatal predictors of postnatal respiratory failure and unique clinical care strategies are discussed. Pulmonary hypoplasia is defined. Historically, fetuses and infants with omphalocele are reported to have markedly reduced chest capacities. Recently, fetal magnetic resonance imaging (MRI) has expanded the understanding of decreased congenital lung volume in infants with omphaloceles. Clinical-radiologic correlation studies support the use of prenatal MRI to predict the degree of respiratory insufficiency observed in the postnatal period.

The contribution of major anomalies to respiratory difficulties is discussed.

Infants with omphalocele may have increased pulmonary vascular reactivity and pulmonary hypertension that increases the postnatal mortality risk. In this chapter, pulmonary hypoplasia and pulmonary hypertension are defined as distinct entities. The chapter emphasizes that the two diagnoses must be distinguished from each other in the clinical setting. Each has different clinical implications and care strategies.

The implications of congenital heart defects in omphalocele infants are explained. The roles and goals of assisted ventilation for respiratory insufficiency in omphalocele infants are expanded.

Since 2011, a small number of infants with omphalocele and respiratory insufficiency have required the extra-corporeal membrane oxygenator (ECMO) for respiratory failure. This chapter provides the first review of the Extra-corporeal Life Support Organization (ELSO, Ann Arbor, MI, USA) database for the causes of respiratory failure and outcomes in omphalocele infants place on ECMO.

The timing of surgical repair and postoperative complications, such as compartment syndrome, delayed surgical closure techniques, and the implications of a ruptured omphalocele, are explained.

Pulmonary function abnormalities, chronic lung disease, the role of tracheostomy, the influence of gastroesophageal reflux disease (GERD), prematurity, and strategies to improve outcomes, are discussed.

2. Giant omphalocele

Giant omphalocele represents an important subset of omphalocele infants. Giant omphalocele is defined as an omphalocele defect containing greater than 75% liver in the sac, and/or a diameter greater than 5 cm [4, 6]. A nongiant omphalocele is generally defined as a defect with diameter less than 5 cm. Previous definitions that measured the defect in centimeters do not account for the differences in size and gestational age of infants.

The definition that giant omphalocele is a defect that contains greater than 75% liver in the sac is preferable and uniform [4]. Giant omphalocele is associated with poor prognosis in many studies. Giant omphalocele is often associated with a greater incidence of respiratory insufficiency, longer ventilator requirements, and an increased incidence of pulmonary hypoplasia and pulmonary hypertension [6, 7].

Infants with giant omphaloceles have significantly more neonatal morbidity. When large and small omphaloceles are compared, the median length of stay (47 vs. 10 days), median age at full enteral feeds (23 vs. 5 days), median duration of mechanical ventilation (23 vs.7 days), and requirement of supplemental oxygen at 30 days of life (88% vs. 27%) are significantly longer for infants with giant omphaloceles [7].

Respiratory failure is the major cause of mortality in infants with giant omphaloceles [8]. In the neonatal period, these infants have significantly more pulmonary hypoplasia and pulmonary hypertension and therefore, more respiratory difficulties [4, 7, 9]. Lung preservation ventilation strategies are emphasized in infants with giant omphaloceles. The overall in-hospital mortality for infants with giant omphaloceles approaches 20% [6].

After the neonatal period, giant omphalocele infants have more chronic lung disease and gastroesophageal reflux. In contrast, small omphaloceles generally have a good prognosis when they are not associated with lethal malformations or congenital syndromes [5].

Most minor defects are closed primarily. Because of the preponderance for respiratory insufficiency in infants with giant omphaloceles, however, there is more controversy regarding closure techniques.

Infants with giant omphaloceles have suboptimal neurodevelopmental outcomes. Their difficult early course frequently includes hypoxia, acidosis, hypotension during delivery, a long duration of mechanical ventilation, infection, and prolonged hospitalization. These factors all compound and play a role in determining neurologic outcomes.

Giant omphalocele survivors tend to have more significant neurodevelopmental delay than children with other congenital anomalies such as congenital diaphragmatic hernia or congenital heart defects. They appear similar in their neurocognitive outcomes to preterm newborns that develop severe bronchopulmonary dysplasia. This further emphasizes the importance of optimal respiratory management and an understanding of the goals of assisted ventilation for infants with giant omphaloceles [6].

3. Pulmonary hypoplasia and the role of fetal magnetic resonance imaging

Lung hypoplasia is defined as insufficient development of pulmonary airways, alveoli, and vessels [10]. Historically, plain chest radiographs of omphalocele infants revealed a narrow thorax and curved ribs. Measures of chest width and lung area were significantly smaller in giant omphalocele infants. Such abnormalities of lung growth may be the result of a deformation sequence in utero. The liver is displaced in giant omphaloceles and so does not mold the thoracic cage [11–13].

Subsequently, prenatal ultrasound was used to calculate observed/expected lung volumes for fetuses. Two-dimensional ultrasound measured the lung-to-thorax ratio and predicted pulmonary hypoplasia. However, some report the assessment as inaccurate [14]. Three-dimensional ultrasound has improved sensitivity in normal amniotic fluid volume but not oligohydramnios [15, 16].

Presently, fetal magnetic resonance imaging studies have established a curve of normal fetal lung volume values plotted against gestational age [17]. The measured fetal lung volume is divided by the expected mean fetal lung volume for a given gestational age or fetal body volume to obtain the observed/expected total fetal lung volume (O/E-TFLV) ratio [17].

Accurate measurement of fetal lung volume has important clinical applications. Fetal magnetic resonance imaging has shown that lung volumes are only 50% of the predicted values in some prematurely born omphalocele infants with large defects. Such infants have lower Apgar scores and require prolonged ventilator support [18].

When infants with congenital lung malformations (CLMs), congenital diaphragmatic hernias (CDHs), or omphaloceles and an O/E-TFLV of 40% to 60% are compared, the need for ECMO, the use of supplemental oxygen at 30 days of life, and the 6-month mortality are similar among the three groups (**Table 1**) [19].

Variable	**CDH** $n = 27$	**Omphalocele** $n = 13$	**CLM** $n = 16$	***p*-value**
Length of intubation, days median (IQR)	9.0 (7–17)	0 (0–6)*	0 (0–1.3)*	<0.001
Length of hospital stay, days median (IQR)	29.0 (22–55)	30.5 (15–47)	8.0 (3–20)*#	0.009

Variable	CDH $n = 27$	Omphalocele $n = 13$	CLM $n = 16$	p-value
Pulmonary HTN, n (%)	11/27 (40.7%)	0/13 (0%)*	0/16 (0%)*	0.001
Treatment of pulmonary HTN n (%)	7/27 (25.9%)	0/13 (0%)	0/16 (0%)*	0.014
iNO utilization n (%)	4/27 (14.8%)	0/13 (0%)	0/16 (0%)	0.099
ECMO n (%)	1/27 (3.7%)	0/13 (0%)	0/16 (0%)	0.579
Supplemental oxygen at 30 DOL n (%)	7/27 (25.9%)	3/13 (23.1%)	1/16 (6.3%)	0.274
Mortality at 6 months n (%)	0/27 (0%)	1/13 (7.7%)	0/16 (0%)	0.234

IQR: interquartile range; HTN: hypertension; iNO: inhaled nitric oxide; ECMO: extra-corporeal membrane oxygenation; supplemental O_2 at 30 DOL: supplemental oxygen at 30 days of life
*$p < 0.05$ vs. CDH.
#$p < 0.05$ vs. OM.

Table 1. Outcomes of congenital diaphragmatic hernia (CDH), omphalocele (OM), and congenital lung malformation (CLM) in infants with fetal lung volumes between 40% and 60% of predicted values [19].

In fetuses with CLM, an O/E-TFLV of less than 75% after 26 weeks predicts a difficult postnatal course that includes increased respiratory distress, a need for intubation, and lung mass excision [20].

Infants with CDH generally have O/E-TFLV measurements ranging from less than 25% to 45%. They require more pulmonary support than omphalocele and congenital lung malformation infants. Clinical-radiologic correlation studies support the use of prenatal MRI to predict the perinatal and postnatal courses in neonates with CDH. The measurements have also been used to guide the fetal therapy with improved postnatal results. Ratios less than 35% are associated with an increased use of ECMO and a higher mortality [21].

A series of infants with giant omphaloceles compare those with less than 50% to infants with greater than 50% O/E-TFLV at 26 to 31 weeks gestational age. Infants with less than 50% O/E-TFLV have significantly lower Apgar scores at birth, prolonged ventilation, and a longer hospitalization. MRI-based O/E-TFLV of less than 50% is considered predictive of increased postnatal morbidity in giant omphalocele infants [18].

A precise quantification of compromised fetal lung development in omphalocele infants may improve perinatal and postnatal management. Fetal magnetic resonance imaging after 26 weeks gestational age and calculation of the O/E-TFLV is recommended.

Similar to CDH and CLM, this calculation reflects pulmonary hypoplasia and allows clinicians to prepare for increased respiratory distress, a need for intubation after birth, and chronic ventilator support. Similar to CDH, further studies may prove that it prognosticates for ECMO use and for mortality. Detailed prenatal counseling and realistic expectations can be provided.

For infants that do not survive, lung-volume-to-body-weight ratios have been established for term and preterm infants [10]. Assessment of lung growth is a critical component of perinatal autopsy. One single series review reports lung biopsy or autopsy pathologic diagnosis of pulmonary hypoplasia or pulmonary hypertension in five omphalocele cases but does not expand on the precise histology details [7].

Fetal magnetic resonance lung volume curves and pathologic lung-volume-to-body-weight ratios for gestational age exist, but clinical-pathologic correlation studies are needed to further characterize pulmonary hypoplasia in infants with omphaloceles.

4. The contribution of major anomalies

Infants with major anomalies and omphaloceles have a longer duration of mechanical ventilation, hospital stay and a need for oxygen at 30 days of life. In a single-institution series of 82 live-born infants, 26% had chromosomal and 30% had major associated anomalies. None of the 19 live-born infants with an isolated defect died. Mortality, however, was 41% and 17% for those with major and minor anomalies, respectively [22].

The presence of associated anomalies is a strong predictor of morbidity and mortality, and anomalies are also linked to respiratory status [5, 16, 23].

Beckwith-Wiedemann syndrome is characterized by omphalocele, macroglossia, macrosomia, hypoglycemia, and embryonic tumors. It is a growth disorder due to dysregulation of the growth regulatory gene on chromosome 11p15 [23]. The presence of hypoglycemia in the perinatal period should alert the clinician to the possibility of Beckwith-Wiedemann syndrome.

The finding of omphalocele on a prenatal ultrasound should prompt a search for associated anomalies and possible further prenatal testing. In a large prenatal study of 445 fetuses with omphalocele, diagnosed in the first trimester, only 55 were live born. Over 85% died in utero due to the presence of fatal chromosomal anomalies [2, 3].

The presence of omphalocele indicates an increased risk of aneuploidy. In a recent first trimester study, fetuses with an omphalocele were found to carry a chromosomal abnormality in 55% of cases [16]. The most frequent abnormal karyotypes in omphalocele infants are Trisomy 18 and 13 [24]. Both have almost 100% incidence of congenital heart defects, including ventricular septal defect, atrial septal defect, and double outlet right ventricle. Infants with omphaloceles, in the setting of Trisomy 13 or 18 and a congenital heart defect, tend to have severe hemodynamic compromise.

http://dx.doi.org/10.5772/63735

In the setting of omphalocele and major anomalies, the cardiopulmonary support provided by the clinician is intensified [25].

Congenital diaphragmatic hernia is sporadically reported in conjunction with an omphalocele. Careful review of fetal MRI of the diaphragm may identify congenital diaphragmatic hernia. Conflicting reports exist, but generally pulmonary hypertension is profound and the outcome is poor [7, 26]. Elevated hemidiaphragms, diaphragmatic eventration, and congenital diaphragmatic hernia have been described in infants with giant omphaloceles, and could contribute to impaired lung development and postnatal distress [8, 11, 27].

5. Pulmonary hypertension

Previously, nonspecific respiratory insufficiency at birth was reported as an independent predictor of mortality for infants with omphaloceles. Older reports do not distinguish between pulmonary hypertension and pulmonary hypoplasia in their contribution to ventilation difficulties.

Pulmonary hypertension is now established as an independent predictor of mortality in infants with omphaloceles [28]. One recent series found that mortality was highest for live-born infants with omphaloceles diagnosed with pulmonary hypertension (45%), considerably higher than mortality in a cohort of infants with omphaloceles alone (18%) [29]. The contribution of pulmonary hypertension to respiratory insufficiency was previously unappreciated [28].

Pulmonary hypertension is diagnosed using echocardiography performed after the second day of life. Changes in the transitional circulation on the first day of life preclude evaluation for pulmonary hypertension by echocardiography. Directionality of flow through the ductus arteriosus is not considered in the diagnosis of pulmonary hypertension on the first day of life.

Pulmonary hypertension is defined on echocardiography as flattening of the interventricular septum during systole and/or a tricuspid regurgitant jet (TR) with an estimated right ventricular pressure greater than 40 mmHg when observed in the setting of hypoxemia [28, 30]. Qualitative measures of right-sided stress, as determined by the cardiologist interpreting the study, contribute to the assessment. These are right ventricular dilation, right atrial enlargement, right ventricular hypertrophy, septal flattening, and pulmonary artery dilation [28, 30, 31].

The incidence of pulmonary hypertension is reported in 37 to 55% of infants with giant omphaloceles. It is more prevalent in infants with additional anomalies [28, 31]. The explanation, whether structural, oxygen tension related, genetic, or some other cause, remains unknown.

Pulmonary hypertension correlates to endpoints of pulmonary insufficiency, including duration of mechanical ventilation, requirement for high-frequency oscillator ventilation, need for tracheostomy, and reliance on oxygen at the time of discharge from neonatal intensive care unit [31].

Conflicting reports exist regarding the prognosis of infants with giant omphaloceles. Some have mild respiratory distress, achieve early feeding and undergo delayed fascial closure with good results [28]. In contrast, others report a high mortality rate in giant omphalocele infants, relating to the predominance of respiratory insufficiency and pulmonary hypertension.

Several retrospective studies suggest that there may be a direct relationship between giant defects and abnormal pulmonary vascular tone. Clinicians should not focus on the defect diameter, but recognize that respiratory insufficiency and pulmonary hypertension are the prognosticators to identify [8, 18, 32].

A recent multicenter retrospective review illustrates the distribution of respiratory insufficiency and pulmonary hypertension in 51 infants with omphalocele (**Figure 1**). All 51 had echocardiography performed between the day of life 2 and 7 [28].

Sixteen infants (31%) had no pulmonary hypertension and no respiratory insufficiency at birth. Of these, 15 survived (94%) and 1 died (6%).

Of the 51 infants (55%), 28 had pulmonary hypertension, and of these, 13 had respiratory insufficiency (46%) while 15 did not (54%).

Of the 51 (39%), 20 infants had respiratory insufficiency at birth without detectable pulmonary hypertension. Six of twenty (30%) were premature infants with a mean gestational age of 31.7 weeks.

Ninety-two percent of mortalities in the cohort were distributed among the infants with pulmonary hypertension, with or without respiratory failure, or respiratory failure without pulmonary hypertension. Of 38 survivors, one that initially presented with respiratory insufficiency, without pulmonary hypertension, progressed to chronic lung disease and required a tracheostomy and a long-term ventilator support. Of the 15 infants with isolated

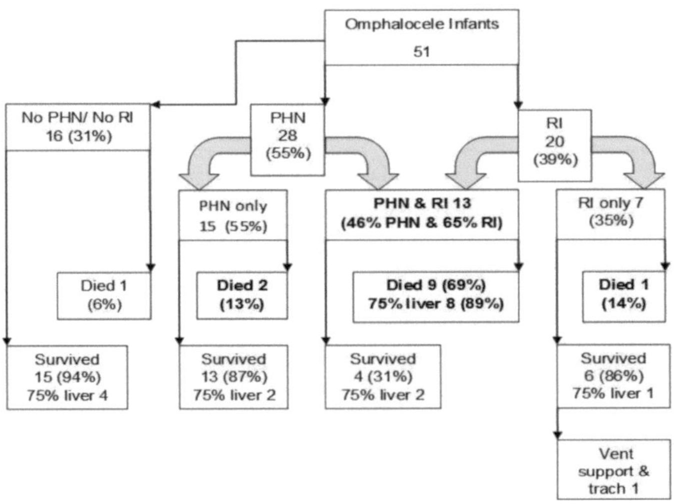

Figure 1. The distribution of respiratory failure and pulmonary hypertension in 51 infants with omphaloceles.

pulmonary hypertension and no evidence of respiratory insufficiency, 13 survived (87%), and none required long-term ventilation (**Figure 1**).

Giant omphalocele defects containing 75% liver were closely associated with mortality. The distribution of 17 giant defects is illustrated among the cohort in **Figure 1**. Eight of seventeen (47%) died, and the eight deaths with giant defects were all distributed in the nine infant deaths that had a combination of pulmonary hypertension and respiratory failure at birth (89%). The distribution of the remaining giant defects is illustrated among the survivors (**Figure 1**) [28].

Logistic regression analysis further revealed that both respiratory insufficiency at birth (OR: 14.8; 95% CI: 2.5–85.0) and pulmonary hypertension diagnosed between days 2 and 7 of life (OR: 6.4; 95% CI: 1.1–39.0) were independently associated with mortality in infants with omphaloceles. This is a new and previously unappreciated finding.

A clinical care strategy that screens for pulmonary hypertension in omphalocele infants is recommended. Echocardiography is best performed between the second and seventh day of life to avoid examination during transitional circulation. Echocardiography should be performed at regular intervals until resolution or stabilization of pulmonary hypertension is demonstrated [28, 30].

The aims of pharmacotherapy for pulmonary hypertension are pulmonary vasodilation, restoration of normal endothelial function, and reversal of remodeling of the pulmonary vasculature. All of these therapies reduce right ventricular afterload and prevent right ventricular failure. Pulmonary vasodilation is needed acutely for pulmonary hypertension, but long-term therapy may focus on vascular remodeling. The main therapies for pulmonary hypertension emphasize the nitric oxide, prostacyclin, and endothelin pathways [33].

There are sporadic reports of the use of ventilator support with inhaled nitric oxide to treat omphalocele infants with pulmonary hypertension. However, detailed reports of lung function measurements before and after trials of inhaled nitric oxide that establish vascular reactivity are few [25]. The phosphodiesterase inhibitor and vasodilator, sildenafil, is administered with success in sporadic series.

After nitric oxide, sildenafil is considered the next-line therapy for pulmonary hypertension in infants, irrespective of etiology [31, 34]. Sildenafil generally improves the oxygenation index with minimal adverse effects in infants with pulmonary hypertension. Despite sildenafil, however, abnormal vascular tone does not necessarily resolve. One-quarter of giant omphalocele infants may require long-term vasodilator therapy with sildenafil [31].

We report one case of giant omphalocele treated with sildenafil and Bosentan. Echo performed at age 4 years shows that the pulmonary hypertension has completely resolved. Bosentan is an oral endothelin receptor antagonist that inhibits vascular remodeling and muscular thickening. Endothelin-1 is believed to play a role in the pathogenesis of neonatal pulmonary hypertension, and endothelin blockade augments pulmonary vasodilation in the perinatal lung. Several reports have shown that Bosentan provides benefit in the treatment of pulmonary hypertension in infants [33].

Selected fetuses may benefit from a maternal hyperoxia study prenatally to predict who will be at risk for elevated pulmonary vascular resistance and pulmonary hypertension, similar to prenatal evaluation in congenital diaphragmatic hernia [25, 35, 36].

The biology of neonatal pulmonary hypertension is linked to lung vascular growth modified by prenatal and early postnatal factors. The use of medical therapy to modify pulmonary hypertension in omphalocele infants is an important area of future study [37].

6. Congenital heart defects

The anterior abdominal wall develops between weeks 3 and 10 of fetal development. The process involves folding of the embryonic disk in cranio-caudal and lateral directions. By week 6 of fetal development, the elongated midgut herniates into the base of the umbilical cord due to lack of space in the abdominal cavity. By the tenth week, it rotates and returns to the abdomen. During this period, the cardiac tubes, which lie on the ventral surface of the embryo, are incorporated into the chest by the lateral folds. Errors in these critical steps of fetal development result in simultaneous anterior abdominal wall defects, such as omphalocele, and structural cardiac defects [25].

In general, a single- or multiinstitutional series of live-born infants with omphaloceles report a 30% incidence of structural congenital heart defects. Neonates with patent ductus arteriosus or patent foramen ovale are not considered to have a congenital heart defect.

A single-center retrospective series found that of 22 live-born omphalocele infants, 7 had evidence of a structural congenital heart defect, 4 of which developed pulmonary hypertension, and 1 of the 4 also had a dysplastic tricuspid valve. Only one infant required a surgical repair, and that infant presented with coarctation of the aorta [25]. The incidence of structural cardiac defects was lower than expected, and this was attributed to the low incidence of abnormal karyotypes.

Another recent multicenter series reports a congenital heart defect incidence in omphalocele infants of 30%, but all were nonductal-dependent lesions without hemodynamic compromise. None had cardiac failure [28].

Although structural cardiac defects should be specifically sought by echo in the first week of life, the influence of congenital heart defects on the outcome for omphalocele infants may be lower than expected, in particular if the cohort has normal karyotypes.

Although clinicians previously evaluated for congenital heart defects, they did not evaluate for pulmonary hypertension. Recent reports clarify that pulmonary hypertension likely has a greater influence on the outcome and mortality in omphalocele infants than congenital heart defects, unless Trisomy 13 or 18 is diagnosed.

In the setting of Trisomy 13 or 18, the incidence of congenital heart defects is over 90%. The most common defects are ventricular septal defect, atrial septal defect, and double outlet right ventricle.

The congenital heart defects of these chromosomal anomalies tend to present with hemodynamic compromise [25, 28, 38]. The establishment of regional and national databases for omphalocele would enhance the statistical understanding of the true incidence of congenital heart defects and hemodynamic compromise in omphalocele infants as few detailed reports with large sample size exist.

7. Respiratory insufficiency and assisted ventilation

Assisted ventilation may be necessary in neonates with omphalocele due to respiratory insufficiency from pulmonary hypoplasia, increased abdominal pressure following surgical repair, diaphragm dysfunction, and pulmonary hypertension [39]. The need for assisted ventilation may occur at delivery or may be confined to the immediate postoperative period related to increased intraabdominal pressure and upward displacement of the diaphragm following closure.

7.1. Goals of assisted ventilation

The goal of assisted ventilation in neonates with respiratory insufficiency due to omphalocele is to achieve adequate functional residual capacity to facilitate gas exchange. Assisted ventilation should be applied to maintain adequate lung volume with even distribution of tidal volume to avoid trauma from atelectasis and lung injury. If lungs with partial atelectasis are ventilated, the tidal volume entering only the open alveoli will lead to overexpansion of the relatively healthy portion of the lung with subsequent trauma due to overexpansion.

Additionally, atelectasis leads to vascular protein leak with increased surfactant inactivation and release of inflammatory mediators. Maintaining adequate lung volume is achieved by applying adequate positive end expiratory pressure (PEEP). There is no single optimal PEEP, and the level must be tailored to the degree of lung injury. For infants with healthy lungs and normal lung compliance, PEEP of 3–4 cm H_2O may be appropriate. Excessive PEEP may lead to overexpansion of normal lungs with circulatory impairment and elevated cerebral venous pressure. However, poorly compliant lungs with atelectasis may transiently require higher PEEP, as high as 8–10 cm H_20 or more, to achieve adequate alveolar recruitment and optimize ventilation/perfusion ratios [40].

For small omphaloceles, if primary abdominal closure has been accomplished, the majority of neonates will require mechanical ventilation for a few days postoperatively. During this time, the abdominal wall and bowel wall edema will improve, and the intraabdominal pressure will decrease.

The elective, routine use of mechanical ventilation to ensure primary closure in every instance is unwarranted. Short-term ventilator support, however, has been a welcomed adjunct to postoperative care and certainly has improved the outlook for these infants [41].

7.2. Noninvasive ventilation

Little information exists regarding the use of continuous positive airway pressure (CPAP) or positive end expiratory pressure (PEEP) in stabilizing the lungs of infants with omphaloceles. Positive end expiratory pressure has been used in premature infants to minimize the effect of excessively compliant chest wall and surfactant deficiency by stabilizing alveoli during the expiratory phase, and has been shown to help establish functional residual capacity.

Traditional management in neonates with omphalocele and respiratory insufficiency involves intubation and mechanical ventilation in the delivery room to presumably avoid further distention of bowel from air swallowing. However, nasal CPAP and/or nasal intermittent positive pressure ventilation may be a preferable approach to improve inadequate respiratory effort in these neonates, while avoiding the complications associated with endotracheal intubation [42].

The noninvasive approach offers the benefit of avoiding an endotracheal tube; therefore, reducing the incidence of ventilator-associated pneumonia and avoiding the contribution of postnatal inflammatory response to the development of bronchopulmonary dysplasia. Noninvasive ventilation reduces iatrogenic lung injury.

7.3. Conventional mechanical ventilation

Several modes of mechanical ventilation have been applied to neonates with omphalocele, but there is little evidence to guide clinicians in selecting the best method. Historically, pressure-controlled ventilation is the standard mode of ventilation in neonates with respiratory failure because of its wide availability, simplicity, ability to ventilate despite large endotracheal tube leak, and improved intrapulmonary gas distribution. However, pressure-controlled ventilation is limited, in that tidal volume varies with changes in lung compliance.

A rapid improvement in compliance may occur in the immediate postnatal period as a result of resorption of lung fluid, recruitment of optimal lung volume, and surfactant replacement therapy, leading to hyperventilation and trauma from excessive lung hyperexpansion [40].

Insufficient tidal volume may develop because of decreasing lung compliance, increasing airway resistance, airway obstruction, air trapping, and/or decreased spontaneous respiratory effort. Inadequate lung volume leads to hypercapnia, increased work of breathing and oxygen consumption, agitation, fatigue and atelectasis/atelectrauma. Low tidal volume leads to inefficient gas exchange due to increased dead space: tidal-volume ratio. Mechanical ventilation goals should include weaning toward extubation, as well as weaning supplemental FiO_2, in order to avoid oxygen toxicity that may contribute to chronic lung disease.

7.4. High-frequency ventilation

In selected infants with respiratory failure due to pulmonary hypoplasia and/or severe pulmonary hypertension, high-frequency ventilation may optimize lung inflation and improve gas exchange. High-frequency ventilation is beneficial as it reduces pressure and volume swings transmitted to the periphery of the lungs, and promotes gentle ventilation. For optimal effectiveness, alveoli must be recruited and stabilized with the lowest possible mean airway pressure.

There is little information in the literature describing the effectiveness of high-frequency ventilation in neonates with omphalocele. In a large single-center series of giant omphalocele infants, mechanical ventilation maintains preductal oxygen saturation above 85% and high-frequency oscillatory ventilation is reserved for patients with refractory hypercapnia [41].

One report examines the use of high-frequency ventilation in 15 omphalocele infants after surgical closure. Of 15 infants, 11 had not required ventilation and were breathing room air prior to operation. High-frequency ventilation is reported as required in six infants (61%) within the first week in the intensive care unit after omphalocele closure. The remainder were managed with conventional ventilation. In half of the 15 infants, lung expansion on chest radiograph was reported at 50%.

The average mean airway pressure at days 5–7 for both the conventional ventilation group and the high-frequency group was 14 mmHg ± 3.0. Weaning from ventilation was achieved on day 7 in only five of the omphalocele infants. Six required ventilation until day 28. Four infants required tracheostomy and prolonged respiratory support between 330 and 1065 days [38]. Prolonged duration of mechanical ventilation and use of parenteral nutrition during this time period likely also contribute to an increased risk of infection.

Primary closure was the procedure of choice in this series. Despite the use of high-frequency ventilation, this series reports a slightly lower survival rate of 73%, compared to the studies with an emphasis on delayed closure that report survival rates of 80% or higher. They note that tension was described by the surgeon in three closures and may have contributed to postoperative difficulties. They note closure of the abdominal wall defect compromised pulmonary mechanics when increased intraabdominal pressure inhibited diaphragmatic movements as the viscera was reduced [38].

This study supports the existence of a degree of pulmonary hypoplasia and decreased pulmonary reserve in omphalocele infants that could only be overcome to a degree by high-frequency ventilation in some but not all of the infants that underwent early closure. It supports the use of delayed closure techniques and careful evaluation of abdominal-visceral disproportion and cardiopulmonary status prior to proceeding with operation [38].

8. Extra-corporeal membrane oxygenation (ECMO)

Despite improvements in the management of respiratory insufficiency and pulmonary hypertension in infants, a number of infants with inadequate gas exchange are treated with extra-corporeal membrane oxygenation (ECMO). This includes infants with omphaloceles.

The authors retrospectively analyzed the Extra-corporeal Life Support Organization (ELSO, Ann Arbor, MI, USA) database between 1992 and 2015 for extra-corporeal membrane oxygenator (ECMO) use and omphalocele. ELSO membership consists of many major medical centers worldwide, with the capability of placing infants on ECMO. This database would capture the majority of infants with omphaloceles, managed with ECMO, during the time period and provide the most of the information about the use of ECMO in these infants. The first infant with an omphalocele was placed on ECMO in 2011.

The specific diagnoses for respiratory insufficiency listed in the database are pulmonary hypertension, congenital heart defects, congenital diaphragmatic hernia, and sepsis. The recorded diagnoses for respiratory insufficiency in the 11 infants were isolated pulmonary hypertension in three; congenital heart defect and pulmonary hypertension in five (one of the five also had capillary alveolar dysplasia); congenital diaphragmatic hernia, congenital heart defect, sepsis, and pulmonary hypertension in one; and congenital diaphragmatic hernia and pulmonary hypertension in two infants.

The six congenital heart defects were double outlet right ventricle in two, Tetralogy of Fallot in one, ventricular septal defect in one, cor triatriatum in one, and aortic atresia/stenosis in one.

Table 2 presents the demographic details and outcomes of 11 infants with omphaloceles placed on ECMO between 2011 and 2015.

	Omphalocele ***N*** **= 11**
First recorded ECMO run	2011
ECMO after day of life 3	8 (73%)
Gender (male)	7 (64%)
Weight at ECMO (kg)[a]	3.27 (2.5–10)
Age at ECMO (days)[a]	10 (0–351)
Run length (hours)[a]	193 (11–589)
A diagnosis of PHN	11 (100%)
Veno-arterial ECMO	10 (91%)
Discontinued from ECMO alive	7 (64%)
Discharged from hospital alive	2 (18%)

Data are expressed in number (%) except with ([a]) data are expressed in median (range).

Table 2. Omphalocele infants that underwent ECMO (2011–2015).

This is a small but significant series as it provides the only data available at present for omphalocele infants and the use of ECMO. The incidence of abnormal karyotypes is not reported with the database, so any association with Trisomy 13 or 18 is unknown.

For infants with omphaloceles that underwent ECMO, between 2011 and 2015 and reported in the ELSO database, the overall mortality was 80%. This high mortality rate contrasts to the reports from a large multicenter series of infants that underwent ECMO for pulmonary hypertension and other conditions such as congenital diaphragmatic hernia between 2000 and 2010, where the mortality rate is 20% or better. These data support the need to better understand the underlying pathophysiology of pulmonary hypertension, so therapy can target its causes in omphalocele infants. There is overlap in the diagnoses of respiratory insufficiency in almost all cases of omphalocele placed on ECMO. Only a large study with multivariate analysis could determine the contribution of each diagnosis to respiratory failure and mortality in omphalocele infants.

One term infant with omphalocele, and respiratory insufficiency attributable to congenital heart defect and pulmonary hypertension, underwent lung biopsy after 10 days of ECMO support. The lung biopsy revealed capillary alveolar dysplasia. Extra-corporeal membrane oxygenation was withdrawn due to the fatal prognosis.

This solitary report raises questions about the etiology of persistent pulmonary hypertension in some omphalocele infants. More autopsy studies and published reports after examination of omphalocele infant lungs may expand the understanding of the contribution of this disorder to pulmonary hypertension and mortality.

Clinically, capillary alveolar dysplasia cannot be distinguished from other syndromes that cause pulmonary hypertension. Histologically, it is characterized by paucity of capillaries adjacent to alveolar epithelium, immature alveolar development, and muscularization of arterioles. The distribution can be diffuse or patchy. The etiology and incidence of capillary alveolar dysplasia are unknown [43].

9. Surgical considerations

The aim of surgical management in infants with omphaloceles is to avoid an abrupt increase in the abdominal pressure that may impair ventilation. An omphalocele which is less than 4 cm in size may be suitable for primary repair after cardiopulmonary stabilization and assessment of anomalies. In contrast, if a giant omphalocele is closed too early, the intraabdominal volume may be insufficient to contain the organs [4, 5].

Immediate postoperative complications are compromise of venous return from a sudden increase in intra-abdominal pressure and cardiopulmonary instability from decreased diaphragmatic excursion. The result is abdominal compartment syndrome (ACS) [38, 39].

Compartment syndrome due to increased intraabdominal pressure is a serious complication after a difficult omphalocele reduction. Early series report a 12% incidence of complications, including acute hepatic congestion, renal failure, and bowel infarction [5, 6].

Before the impact of viscero-abdominal disproportion (VAD) and abdominal compartment syndrome was understood, surgeons placed emphasis on operative closure. Between 1980 and 1995, in a series of 30 operative closures, about half were small defects and were closed primarily without complications [44].

The remainder were giant omphaloceles. Three underwent skin closure due to viscero-abdominal disproportion. Thirteen underwent silo placement and were closed between 11 and

Complication	N (%)
Wound dehiscence	7 (24%)
Gastroesophageal reflux	5 (17%)
Hepatic hematoma	3 (10%)
Hepatic congestion	2 (6%)
Enterocutaneous fistula	2 (6%)
Bowel infarction	1 (3%)
Renal failure	1 (3%)

Table 3. Operative complications [44].

137 days. There were 14 serious complications in 13 infants. All were due to initial tight closure, and all were opened postoperatively. There was one postoperative death (**Table 3**).

No randomized studies show that intraabdominal pressure monitoring is beneficial, and therefore it is not used to guide closure in the operating room, but may have a role in the postoperative period. Continuous bladder pressure monitoring in the postoperative period does not prevent necrotizing enterocolitis, but maintaining abdominal pressure below 20 mmHg prevents renal failure [45].

Various closure techniques for giant omphalocele exist, including alloderm patch, vacuum-assisted closure, tissue expanders, silos, and other types of mesh materials [46, 47]. If the sac is intact, application of topical agents and dressing changes for initial nonoperative management of a giant omphalocele is recommended. This technique transitions to delayed closure [26]. Tension and intraabdominal compression increase morbidity and must be avoided during closure. If tension exists, then a silo or mesh must be used for coverage [38].

In two recent series, infants with giant omphaloceles underwent treatment of the sac with topical agents and delayed closure. The median age of repair was 10 months (range: 3.4–23.6 months) in one series and 215 days in the other. No repairs were opened postoperatively [4, 22]. Six-month survival was 80% in both the series, despite the fact that half of the delayed closure infants in one series met the criteria for pulmonary hypoplasia on fetal magnetic resonance imaging [22].

A recent series of 16 infants with giant omphaloceles achieved discharge and returned for delayed closure during an elective admission at a median of 14 months (range: 2–28 months). The median length of hospital stay for this elective admission was 4 days (range: 2–21 days). One of sixteen (6%) required unexpected prolonged ventilation and stayed in hospital for 21 days. Four (25%) required mesh as viscero-abdominal disproportion had not resolved [26].

When compared to the reports obtained from previous decades, surgeons wait 7–24 months longer before attempting closure of a giant omphalocele. Although no comparative studies exist, the concept of giant omphalocele closure has evolved over the last two decades [38, 39].

Most surgeons promote application of topical agents to the sac, followed by delayed closure. This approach allows improved respiratory status, fewer complications, and better outcomes

[1, 4, 22, 26]. The emphasis on closure has been replaced by a better appreciation of viscero-abdominal disproportion, abdominal compartment syndrome, and the connection between stable cardiopulmonary status and survival.

Clinicians should be aware, however, that even if closure succeeds, a 40–50% reduction in respiratory system compliance on the first and second postoperative days after closure of abdominal wall defects has been demonstrated, as well as a 38% reduction in forced vital capacity.

Mechanical ventilation, including high-frequency ventilation, may be required after delayed omphalocele closure [9, 26, 27].

9.1. Technique of delayed repair

After birth, the application of topical povidone-iodine, silver sulfadiazine or bacitracin ointment and xeroform gauze to the omphalocele sac allows epithelialization. Epithelialization often occurs within 10 weeks [16]. During this time, the infant can begin intestinal feeding.

As the giant omphalocele infant grows, the viscero-abdominal disproportion gradually resolves, but the infant must be clinically monitored. Giant omphalocele infants with respiratory distress, pulmonary hypoplasia, pulmonary hypertension, or sepsis will require specific care strategies, until they meet the criteria for extubation. Surgical closure of the abdominal fascia is not a priority during this time period.

The respiratory status of some giant omphalocele infants improves to the point that they can be discharged, followed as an outpatient, and can return for elective closure [26]. When the omphalocele contents reduce manually into the abdominal cavity with ease, the body cavity is considered large enough to proceed with operative closure.

If the contents fit, the impact on venous return, renal perfusion, and diaphragmatic excursion is decreased. After operative closure, the majority of infants are extubated postoperatively, and the average length of hospital stay is 4 days. A minority of infants may have a longer ventilator time after closure (up to 21 days), and this can be difficult to predict [4, 26]. Parents should be informed of this possibility.

9.2. Ruptured omphalocele

A ruptured omphalocele is defined as any disruption of the omphalocele sac membrane [48]. Rupture of the omphalocele sac is frequently reported as a poor prognosticator associated with sepsis and mortality. The goal of the pediatric surgeon is to cover the eviscerated organs.

Although disrupted, if enough sac exists, it can be successfully sutured together with absorbable sutures.

Successful reduction and coverage of a giant ruptured omphalocele are reported after silo placement and coverage with an absorbable mesh, followed by split thickness skin grafting [49]. Despite coverage, many infants die of respiratory insufficiency and infection [28].

A ruptured sac requires urgent surgical intervention, but only sporadic case reports exist that pertain to specific surgical management of a ruptured omphalocele.

Hemodynamic instability dominates the clinical course in infants with ruptured omphalocele. The majority of infants with ruptured omphalocele require at least 80 ml^{-1} kg^{-1} volume expansion in the first 7 days of life [38]. Intestinal exposure results in increased water and heat loss. Manipulation and closure can result in losses into a third space that exacerbates hypovolemia.

Volume expansion to achieve a mean arterial pressure of 45 mmHg increases blood pressure and urine output. The use of renal dose dopamine is controversial, and benefits have not been confirmed in recent meta-analyses. High-dose norepinephrine should be avoided as it can exacerbate bowel ischemia and necrosis [38].

An infant with ruptured omphalocele requires surgical consultation to obtain organ coverage, but intensive cardiopulmonary support with features of sepsis and a high mortality rate will dominate the clinical course. The association between ruptured omphalocele, sepsis, and mortality is not well understood.

10. Long-term respiratory support

There is a potential need for ongoing mechanical ventilatory support after the neonatal period in neonates born with a giant omphalocele. Partridge observed high rates of reactive airways disease in giant omphalocele survivors that was significantly associated with pulmonary hypertension [31]. Neonates with giant omphalocele and pulmonary hypertension required increased respiratory support based on the significant increases in the duration of mechanical ventilation, requirement for high-frequency oscillatory ventilation and tracheostomy, with dependence on home oxygen therapy following hospital discharge [31].

Whether reactive airways disease is an innate characteristic of the airways of infants with pulmonary hypoplasia associated with giant omphalocele versus increased respiratory support requirements and sequelae of mechanical ventilation remains unclear.

Pulmonary function abnormalities have been described in giant omphalocele survivors, and include reduced mean forced vital capacity and forced expiratory volume on pulmonary function testing with significant bronchodilator responsiveness in almost half of all patients studied [31]. Long-term respiratory issues in infants with giant omphaloceles include asthma, recurrent infections, chronic lung disease, and bronchomalacia.

Prolonged respiratory insufficiency is a frequent complication of giant omphalocele and the major prognostic factor for infants without life-threatening malformations. Infants with giant omphaloceles may require support for respiratory insufficiency into their second year of life. This possibility should be discussed with their families.

Of 22 long-term survivors with giant omphaloceles in a prospective follow-up series, chronic lung disease exists in 40%, and 16% have a tracheostomy for prolonged ventilation at a mean

http://dx.doi.org/10.5772/63735

day of life 154 (median: 156 days; range: 100–204 days) [6]. Of six long-term survivors in a single retrospective series at 33.2 months (range: 20–70 months), three have asthma requiring medical therapy, two have recurrent infections, and one requires overnight continuous positive airway pressure (CPAP) at 20 months for bronchomalacia [4].

Not much data are reported about the indications of tracheostomy in neonates with giant omphalocele, although most retrospective series report a subset that required prolonged ventilation and tracheostomy placement, in general, 5–10% of infants in a series. In general, tracheostomies are placed to secure a safe airway for infants with protracted mechanical ventilation. The optimal timing for tracheostomy placement in these babies is unknown; however, severity of lung disease and problems of airway that preclude extubation are the most common indications.

There is no good evidence for deferring tracheostomy because infants are receiving high ventilator pressures. While high ventilator settings may be a concern that discourages consideration of tracheostomy placement, appropriate developmental interventions are nearly impossible to implement without placement of a tracheostomy in infants with an unstable artificial airway [50].

11. Gastroesophageal reflux disease (GERD)

In infants with omphaloceles, the incidence of gastroesophageal reflux disease (GERD) with associated esophagitis approaches 45% [51]. Gastroesophageal reflux disease is diagnosed at a median age of 7 months and is more prevalent in infants with giant defects. Infants with omphalocele and a large defect have a high incidence of GERD complicated by esophagitis during the first few years of life [51].

Frequently, the retrospective series reports infants with omphaloceles and GERD that fail medical therapy and undergo Nissen fundoplication [6].

Pulmonary function studies were performed on follow-up of 30 giant omphalocele infants at a median of 19 months. The studies performed were spirometry, fractional lung volume measurements, assessment of bronchodilator responsiveness and passive respiratory mechanics, to evaluate the nature and degree of pulmonary dysfunction in these survivors. The series reports lung volume restriction without obstruction, an increased likelihood of airway hyperresponsiveness and reduced compliance in almost 50% of the infants studied [31, 52]. Early recognition of pulmonary functional impairment may help develop targeted treatment strategies for these infants, and this may include evaluation and treatment for GERD.

Partridge reports similar high rates of reactive airways disease in giant omphalocele survivors. Follow-up pulmonary function study results are similar to those obtained for infants with congenital diaphragmatic hernia and bronchopulmonary dysplasia. There may be a common etiology between pulmonary hypoplasia and reactive airways disease. The same series of omphalocele infants also reports a 10% rate of Nissen fundoplication for symptomatic GERD.

Targeted treatment strategies are not well established, but GERD will exacerbate hyperactive airways and asthma. Evidence for GERD should be sought by pH probe studies or endoscopy to diagnose esophagitis in infants with omphaloceles. Contrast radiographs may also add information regarding the esophageal-gastric anatomy and the presence of GERD. Any contribution of GERD to airway responsiveness should decrease with appropriate medical and/or surgical therapy.

12. Prematurity

In the majority of series that examine outcomes in omphalocele infants and factors associated with mortality, when factors such as respiratory insufficiency, pulmonary hypertension, and measures of pulmonary hypoplasia are examined, the influence of prematurity (defined as an infant born before 37 weeks gestation) is rarely as preponderant as other respiratory comorbidities. In the first series that reported respiratory insufficiency as an independent predictor of mortality in omphalocele infants, respiratory insufficiency at birth was found to be independent of gestational age [1].

In a recent multicenter series of 51 infants that found pulmonary hypertension and respiratory insufficiency at birth were associated with mortality in omphalocele infants, the median gestational age was 38.2 weeks (range: 28.0–40.0 weeks) for survivors and 34.6 weeks (range: 29.0–40.4 weeks) for mortalities [28]. There was no significant difference in gestational age between survivors and nonsurvivors. Respiratory insufficiency and pulmonary hypertension were associated with mortality, independent of gestational age. Of seven infants with respiratory insufficiency at birth, but without evidence of pulmonary hypertension, six survived. None of the remaining 44 infants in the series were premature. There was no significant association between prematurity, respiratory insufficiency, and mortality that could be identified in these infants with omphaloceles [28].

In contrast, in one study from Porter, preterm birth complicated more than a third of omphalocele cases, and the only neonatal deaths occurred because of complications of prematurity [53]. This is an isolated report.

Another series reports that the presence of major anomalies was the most significant factor associated with pulmonary morbidity, independent of gestational age [19].

For the majority of series that examine the influence of various factors on respiratory insufficiency, morbidity, and mortality in omphalocele infants, the influence of prematurity is not as predominant as other factors. This is likely because the median gestational age for most series is closer to term as modern prenatal care and monitoring of high-risk pregnancies may prevent preterm birth. For infants that are premature, if there is no pulmonary hypertension or pulmonary hypoplasia, the modern neonatal care of premature infant lungs is now sophisticated to the point that an influence on mortality cannot be consistently identified in the retrospective series.

13. Conclusions

Despite advances in neonatal care, mortality rates for infants with omphaloceles remain between 5% and 25% [4]. In this chapter, the unique aspects of respiratory management in omphalocele infants and care strategies are discussed. The chapter emphasizes pulmonary hypoplasia as distinct from pulmonary hypertension. Pulmonary hypoplasia is defined as insufficient development of pulmonary airways, alveoli, and vessels. Fetal MRI after 26 weeks gestational age with calculation of the O/E-TFLV is recommended. A prenatal O/E-TFLV of less than 50% predicts lower Apgar scores and a longer duration of mechanical ventilation. It may eventually prognosticate for mortality.

Pulmonary hypertension is an independent predictor of mortality in omphalocele infants [28]. A relationship may exist between giant defects and abnormal pulmonary vascular tone. Respiratory insufficiency and pulmonary hypertension, not the defect diameter, are the prognosticators to identify [8, 18, 32]. We recommend echocardiography between days 2 and 7 of life to evaluate for pulmonary hypertension. After diagnosis, echocardiography should be performed at regular intervals, until stabilization is demonstrated [28, 30].

Assisted-ventilation concepts in omphalocele infants are similar for all neonates with respiratory compromise. Gentle ventilation, adequate gas exchange, and early extubation minimize adverse outcomes. A longer duration of ventilation is associated with chronic lung disease, sepsis, and neurodevelopmental impairment [6]. Infants with giant omphaloceles represent a subgroup that benefit from these concepts. They frequently have several comorbidities and a longer period of respiratory insufficiency after birth.

Review of the ELSO database reveals that for infants with omphaloceles requiring ECMO, between 2011 and 2015, the mortality is estimated at 80%. Clinicians should consider these results before recommending ECMO. The surgical approach for infants with omphaloceles has evolved over the last two decades. The emphasis on primary closure is now replaced by an appreciation of viscero-abdominal disproportion and abdominal compartment syndrome [1, 4, 22, 26].

Respiratory management for infants with omphaloceles may be arduous. Application of specific definitions allows targeting of therapy and clinical strategies. A multidisciplinary approach by perinatology, pediatric surgery, and neonatology may allow comprehensive evaluation of respiratory status. Analysis of prenatal information followed by postnatal clinical correlation may improve the outcomes for infants with omphaloceles.

Acknowledgements

The authors thank Douglas Deming, MD, for reviewing the manuscript.

Author details

Joanne Baerg*, Arul Thirumoorthi and Andrew Hopper

*Address all correspondence to: jbaerg@llu.edu

Loma Linda University Children's Hospital, Loma Linda, CA, USA

References

[1] Tsakayannis DE, Zurakowski D, Lillehei CW. Respiratory insufficiency at birth: A predictor of mortality for infants and omphalocele. J Pediatr Surg 1996;31:1088–91.

[2] Tassin M, Descriaud C, Elie C, et al. Omphalocele in the first trimester: Prediction of perinatal outcome. Prenat Diagn 2013;33:497–501.

[3] Brantberg A, Blaas HG, Haugen SE, Eik-Nes SH. Characteristics and outcome of 90 cases of fetal omphalocele. Ultrasound Obstet Gynecol 2005;26:527–37.

[4] Biard JM, Douglas Wilson R, Johnson MP, et al. Prenatally diagnosed omphaloceles: Short and long-term outcomes. Prenat Diagn 2004;24:434–9.

[5] Mcnair C, Hawes J, Urquhart H. Caring for the newborn with an omphalocele. Neonatal Netw 2006;25:319–27.

[6] Danzer E, Gerdes M, D'Agostino JA, et al. Prospective interdisciplinary follow-up of children with prenatally diagnosed giant omphalocele: Short-term neurodevelopmental outcome. J Pediatr Surg 2010;45:718–23.

[7] Vachharajani AJ, Rao R, Keswani S, Mathur AM. Outcomes in exomphalos: An institutional experience. Pediatr Surg Int 2009;25:139–44.

[8] Edwards EA, Broome S, Green S, et al. Long-term respiratory support in children with giant omphalocele. Anaesth Intensive Care 2007;35:94–8.

[9] Dimitriou G, Greenough A, Giffin F, et al. Temporary impairment of lung function in infants with anterior abdominal wall defects who have undergone surgery. J Pediatr Surg 1996;31:670–2.

[10] De Paepe ME, Shapiro S, Hansen K, Gundogan F. Postmortem lung volume/body weight standards for term and preterm infants. Pediatr Pulmonol 2014;49:60–6.

[11] Hershenson MB, Brouillette RT, Klemka I, et al. Respiratory insufficiency in newborns with abdominal wall defects. J Pediatr Surg 1985;20:348–53.

[12] Griscom NT, Driscoll SG. Radiography of stillborn fetuses and infants dying at birth. AJR Am J Roentgenol 1980;134:485–9.

[13] Argyle JC. Pulmonary hypoplasia in infants with giant abdominal wall defects. Pediatr Pathol 1989;9:43–55.

[14] Kamata S, Usul N, Sawai T, Nose K, Fukuawa M. Prenatal detection of pulmonary hypoplasia in giant omphalocele. Pediatr Surg Int 2008;24:107–11.

[15] Prendergast M, Rafferty GF, Davenport M, et al. Three-dimensional ultrasound fetal lung volumes and infant respiratory outcome: A prospective observational study. BJOG 2011;118:608–14.

[16] Prefumo F, Izzi C. Fetal abdominal wall defects. Best Pract Res Clin Obstet Gynaecol 2014;28:391–402.

[17] Rypens F, Metens T, Rocourt N, et al. Fetal lung volume: Estimation at MR imaging—initial results. Radiology 2001;219:236–41.

[18] Danzer E, Victoria T, Bebbington MW, et al. Fetal MRI calculated total lung volumes in the prediction of short-term outcome in giant omphalocele: Preliminary findings. Fetal Diagn Ther 2012;31:248–53.

[19] Akinkuotu AC, Sheikh F, Cass DL, et al. Are all pulmonary hypoplasias the same? A comparison of pulmonary outcomes in neonates with congenital diaphragmatic hernia, omphalocele and congenital lung malformation. J Pediatr Surg 2015;50:55–9.

[20] Zamora I, Sheikh F, Cassady C. Fetal MRI lung volumes are predictive of perinatal outcomes in fetuses with congenital lung masses. J Pediatr Surg. 2014;49:853–8.

[21] Akinkuotu A, Cruz S, Abbas P, et al. Risk stratification for infants with CDH: Prenatal vs. postnatal predictors of outcome. J Pediatr Surg 2016;51:44–8.

[22] Akinkuotu A, Sheikh F, Olutuye O, et al. Giant omphaloceles: Surgical management and perinatal outcomes. J Surg Res 2015;198:388–92.

[23] Chen CP. Syndromes and disorders associated with omphalocele. Taiwan J Obstet Gynecol 2007;46:96–102.

[24] Khalil A, Arnaoutoglou C, Pacilli M, et al. Outcome of fetal exomphalos diagnosed at 11-14 weeks gestation. Ultrasound Obstet Gynecol 2012;39:401–6.

[25] Gibbin C, Touch S, Groth R, Berghella V. Abdominal wall defects and congenital heart disease. Ultrasound Obstet Gynecol 2003;21:334–7.

[26] Lee SL, Beyer TD, Kim SS, et al. Initial nonoperative management and delayed closure for treatment of infants with giant omphaloceles. J Pediatr Surg 2006;41:1846–9.

[27] Nakayama DK, Mutich R, Motoyama EK. Pulmonary dysfunction after primary closure of an abdominal wall defect and its improvement with bronchodilators. Pediatr Pulmonol 1992;12:174–80.

[28] Baerg JE, Thorpe DL, Sharp NE, et al. Pulmonary hypertension predicts mortality in infants with omphalocele. J Neonatal Perinat Med 2016;8:333–8.

[29] Corey K, Hornik C, Laughon M, et al. Frequency of anomalies and hospital outcomes in infants with gastroschisis and omphalocele. Early Hum Dev 2014;90:421–4.

[30] Mourani P, Sontag M, Younoszai A, et al. Clinical utility of echocardiography for the diagnosis and management of pulmonary vascular disease in young children with chronic lung disease. Pediatrics 2008;121:317–25.

[31] Partridge EA, Hanna BD, Panitch HB, et al. Pulmonary hypertension in giant omphalocele infants. J Pediatr Surg 2014;49:1767–70.

[32] van Eijck FC, Hoogeveen YL, van Weel C, et al. Minor and giant omphalocele: Long-term outcomes and quality of life. J Pediatr Surg 2009;44:1355–9.

[33] Steinhorn, RH. Diagnosis and treatment of pulmonary hypertension in infancy. Early Hum Dev 2013;89:865–74.

[34] Archer SL, Michelakis ED. An evidence-based approach to the management of pulmonary areterial hypertension. Curr Opin Cardiol 2006;21;385–92.

[35] Rasanen J, Wood DC, Debbs R, et al. Reactivity of the human fetal circulation to maternal hyperoxygenation increases in the second half of pregnancy, a randomized study. Circulation 1998;97:257–62.

[36] Broth RE, Wood DC, Rasanen J, et al. Prenatal prediction of lethal pulmonary hypoplasia: The hyperoxygenation test for pulmonary artery reactivity. Am J Obstet Gynecol 2002;187:940–5.

[37] Abman S, Baker C, Gien J, et al. The Robyn Barst memorial lecture: Differences between fetal, newborn, and adult pulmonary circulations: Relevance for age-specific therapies. Pulm Circ 2014;4:424–40.

[38] Aizenfisz S, Dauger S, Gondon E, et al. Gastroschisis and omphalocele: Retrospective study of initial postoperative management in the ICU. Eur J Pediatr Surg 2006;16:84–9.

[39] Panitch H. Pulmonary complications of abdominal wall defects. Pediatr Resp Rev 2015;16:11–7.

[40] Kezler M, Gizzi SA. Mechanical ventilation and bronchopulmonary dysplasia. Bronchopulmonary dysplasia: An update. Clin Perinatol 2015;42:781–96.

[41] Christison-Lagay ER, Kelleher CM, Langer JC. Neonatal abdominal wall defects. Semin Fetal Neonatal Med 2011;16:164–72.

[42] Moretti C, Gizzi C, Papoff P et al. Comparing the effects of nasal synchronized intermittent positive pressure ventilation (nSIPPV) and nasal continuous positive airway pressure (nCPAP) after extubation in very low birth weight infants. Early Hum Dev 1999;56:167–77.

[43] Gerrits LC, De Mol AC, Bulten J, Van der Staak FH, Van Heijst AF. Omphalocele and alveolar capillary dysplasia: A new association. Pediatr Crit Care Med 2010;11:36–7.

[44] Dunn J, Fonkalsrud E. Improved survival in infants with omphalocele. Am J Surg 1997;173:284–7.

[45] Engum SA, Kogon B, Jensen E, et al. Gastric tonometry and direct intraabdominal pressure measuring in abdominal compartment syndrome. J Pediatr Surg. 2002;37:214–8.

[46] Binet A, Gelas T, Jochault-Ritz S, et al. VAC therapy a therapeutic alternative in giant omphalocele treatment: A multicenter study. J Plast Reconstr Aesthet Surg 2013;66:373–5.

[47] Barkat A, Shetty A, McKee J. A novel approach for the closure of challenging giant omphalocele. J Pediatr Surg Case Rep 2015;3:485–8.

[48] Ledbetter DJ. Congenital abdominal wall defects and reconstruction in pediatric surgery: Gastroschisis and omphalocele. Surg Clin North Am 2012;92(3):713–27.

[49] Yamagishi J, Takayasu H, Otani Y, et al. Visceral coverage with absorbable mesh followed by split-thickness skin graft in the treatment of ruptured giant omphalocele. Pediatr Surg Int 2007;23:199–201.

[50] Mandy G, Malkar M, Welty SE, et al. Tracheostomy placement in infants with bronchopulmonary dysplasia: Safety and outcomes Pediatr Pulmonol 2013;48:245–9.

[51] Koivusalo A, Rintala R, Lindahl H. Gastroesophageal reflux in children with congenital abdominal wall defects. J Pediatr Surg 1999;34:1127–9.

[52] Danzer E, Hedrick H, Rintoul N, et al. Assessment of early pulmonary function abnormalities in giant omphalocele survivors. J Pediatr Surg 2012;47:1811–20.

[53] Porter A, Benson CB, Hawley P, et al. Outcome of fetuses with a prenatal ultrasound diagnosis of isolated omphalocele. Prenat Diag 2009;29:668–73.

Chapter 4

Respiratory Care Protocols in Neonatal Intensive Care

Wissam Shalish and Guilherme Mendes Sant' Anna

Additional information is available at the end of the chapter

http://dx.doi.org/10.5772/63556

Abstract

Neonatal respiratory care involves physicians with variable backgrounds treating multiple respiratory problems and populations with a number of invasive and non-invasive devices and strategies. Unfortunately, there is a lack of strong evidence to guide the most adequate management for several specific situations. Altogether, this complexity leads to significant practice variability that can affect patient and health care outcomes. Respiratory care protocols, guided by evidence and/or consensus, are an attractive solution to promote standardization of care and reduction of unnecessary practice variations. Indeed, despite the limited evidence supporting the use of respiratory protocols in neonates, a significant number of units have already developed and implemented them into clinical practice. Respiratory care protocols appear to promote evidence-based practices, discourage outdated approaches and ultimately improve patient safety.

Keywords: neonates, protocols, respiratory support, mechanical ventilation, intensive care

1. Introduction

The hallmark of neonatology relies on adequate provision of respiratory care, most commonly in the form of noninvasive respiratory support or mechanical ventilation (MV). Also, adjunctive therapies such as surfactant, caffeine, postnatal steroids and inhaled nitric oxide play important roles. In the past decade, a large number of strategies to guide respiratory care practices have been investigated in an attempt to improve neonatal short- and long-term outcomes, including length of MV, extubation failure rates, bronchopulmonary dysplasia (BPD) and neurodevelopment. Unfortunately, there is often limited or conflicting evidence to guide clinicians, leading to highly variable practices and a wide display of outcomes across neonatal intensive care units (NICUs). One way to decrease unnecessary variations in practice is through the use of clinical protocols. The objective of this chapter is to (1) describe the variability of respiratory care practices in neonatology; (2) evaluate the impact of practice variability on patient and health care outcomes; (3) review the evidence for using respiratory care protocols in neonates; and (4) provide an overview on how to develop and implement these protocols in the NICU.

2. Variability of respiratory care practices in neonatology

In the modern era of neonatology, with the introduction of many new technologies and adjunctive therapies, the provision of adequate respiratory care has become very complex and challenging. Several local, national and international surveys have been undertaken to describe how these therapies are utilized across NICUs, consistently revealing wide intra- and inter-center variability.

2.1. Respiratory care management in the delivery room

Approximately 10% of neonates require some degree of respiratory assistance after birth [1]. As an inadequate delivery of respiratory support may have serious repercussions, it is crucial for health care providers to have a solid foundation in neonatal resuscitation while staying up-to-date with recent advances in the field. A number of national and international expert consortiums regularly publish evidence-based guidelines to help providers during this critical period [1]. Despite these recommendations, surveys from around the world continue to demonstrate wide variations in many aspects of respiratory care management in the delivery room.

The most striking illustration of variability is ventilation during neonatal resuscitation. Units provide positive pressure ventilation using various methods, including the flow-inflating bag (2–63%), self-inflating bag (6–96%), T-piece/Neopuff (1–79%) and ventilator (16–49%) [2–9]. These can be delivered via face mask, binasal prongs, single nasal prong or a nasopharyngeal tube. Many institutions have more than one device at their disposal. Although positive-end-expiratory pressure (PEEP) is now commonly used during positive pressure ventilation, many centers that use the self-inflating bag do not apply it with a PEEP valve or manometer [6]. In addition, delivered peak inflation pressures vary with regard to the maximal level and duration of the inflation [5, 8]. Continuous positive airway pressure (CPAP) in the delivery room has gained popularity over the past years, particularly for the preterm population. But its use varies between 50 and 85% across countries, with units setting different gestational age thresholds (anywhere from 24–32 weeks) above which they would attempt CPAP [2, 3, 5, 9]. For those infants who get intubated, 3–45% of units have reported using CO_2 detectors [4, 6–9]. Moreover, there are variations in the preferred routes of intubation (oral vs. nasal) and types of endotracheal tubes used (straight vs. shouldered) [5].

The second most prominent source of variability in the delivery room relates to oxygenation. Despite evidence-based recommendations on the use of pulse oximetry (PO), oxygen blenders and resuscitation of term infants with room air [1], some units have not yet adopted these practices. Routine use of PO and O_2 blenders ranges from 30 to 100% and 36 to 100% across units, respectively [2, 5–10]. Although guidelines recommend preductal saturation measurements, one survey showed that only 37% of units placed their saturation probes correctly [3]. Similarly, 7–56% of units have been reported to initiate resuscitation in 100% oxygen [3, 4, 7, 10]. In the case of preterm infants, the starting concentration of oxygen varies considerably (between 21 and 100%), with some providers starting high and tapering down and others doing the contrary [8]. Oxygen is commonly titrated based on predefined oxygen saturation targets, but some units still adjust according to color and heart rate [6].

2.2. Invasive mechanical ventilation

With the rapid advent of technology, clinicians can now choose from a wide range of ventilators and modalities for invasive MV. Some surveys have reported as many as 12 different brands of ventilators for delivering conventional MV and at least 4 different types of machines for providing high-frequency oscillatory ventilation (HFOV), with many units having more than one type at their disposal [11–13]. There are currently over 10 different MV modes available, including assist control (pressure or volume controlled), intermittent mandatory ventilation (with or without synchronization, with or without pressure support), HFOV (with or without volume control), high-frequency jet ventilation and neurally adjusted ventilatory assist (NAVA). Use of all these ventilators and modalities is rarely guided by patient disease or best evidence, but rather by availability, familiarity and personal preferences [11–16].

A noticeable observation from recent surveys reveals that volume-targeted ventilation has yet to gain widespread adoption during MV, despite established evidence for its use as a lung-protective strategy [17]. There are significant geographical variations in volume-targeted ventilation use, ranging from 5 to 60% [12–14, 16, 18, 19]. With regard to the preset tidal volume (V_T), the recommended target is generally 4–7ml/kg. However, surveys have demonstrated that some units use V_T targets as low as 3–4ml/kg and as high as 10ml/kg [18, 19]. Another prospective observational study showed that as many as 18% of units used V_T levels higher than 7ml/kg [12]. These extremes of low and excessive V_T may predispose to inadequate ventilation and volutrauma, respectively.

Furthermore, tools used for monitoring and titrating MV settings are quite heterogeneous. For instance, gas exchange can be monitored using $PaCO_2$ levels in the blood, transcutaneous CO_2, end tidal CO_2 or near-infrared spectroscopy [16, 20]. There is generally no consensus on the blood gas route (venous, arterial or capillary), frequency of sampling and thresholds for titrating. Although some evidence suggests that permissive hypercapnia may be a lung-protective strategy during MV, a recent survey in the USA showed that clinicians aimed for various target PCO_2 levels, anywhere between 45 and 65 mmHg [21]. Ventilator settings are also titrated in many different ways. In one Canadian survey, PEEP could be titrated on the basis of oxygen saturation, pulse oximetry, blood gas, fraction of inspired oxygen (FiO_2) or chest x-ray findings [16]. The indications and frequency of performing chest x-rays in intubated neonates are also rarely delineated and subject to individual preferences.

There are many other aspects of MV that lend themselves to practice inconsistencies. Endotracheal tubes (ETTs) are secured using various taping methods. Infants are suctioned via the ETT at different frequencies and techniques. Practices relating to infant positioning (supine vs. prone) or the ability to do kangaroo care during MV are also nurse or clinician dependent. Most importantly, the use of sedation during MV is so controversial that it has led to very changeable practices; some clinicians always provide opiates and/or sedatives to intubated patients, while others sometimes or never use it [14, 15].

2.3. Peri-extubation practices

In order to limit complications associated with MV, infants are often extubated as early as possible. The process of extubation is quite complex and consists of three important steps: weaning from MV, assessment of extubation readiness and provision of post-extubation respiratory support. Significant variations in practice exist for all components of this process, with decisions often being physician dependent and not always evidence based. For instance, synchronized intermittent mandatory ventilation (SIMV) appears to be the most commonly used weaning mode across surveys [13, 14, 16], despite the evidence that assist control ventilation confers more homogeneous V_T and faster weaning when compared to SIMV [22]. Furthermore, in a recent international survey focused on extremely preterm infants, extubation readiness was primarily assessed based on the subjective interpretation of ventilator settings, blood gases and overall clinical stability [23]. In addition, 16% of infants were extubated infants on the basis of passing a spontaneous breathing trial, although the trial was often conducted in variable ways. The timing of extubation was extremely variable, with some units removing the ETT immediately after surfactant administration while others only after 2 weeks of MV. Finally, 10% of the centers still reported extubating extremely preterm infants to low-flow nasal cannula, oxyhood or no respiratory support despite the undisputed evidence favoring the use of noninvasive ventilation in this population [24].

2.4. Noninvasive ventilation

Continuous positive airway pressure—Since its discovery in the late 1970s, CPAP has been extensively studied in neonates. Consequently, it is by far the most widely used noninvasive mode across the world. Although CPAP has been well established and widely adopted for the treatment of apnea of prematurity and following extubation of preterm infants, its use as a primary therapy for respiratory distress syndrome (RDS) has only recently gained attraction. A recent study comparing epidemiological data from the Vermont Oxford and Italian Neonatal Networks revealed significantly high coefficients of variation in the use of CPAP as a primary therapy, ranging from 0 to 80% [25]. To provide CPAP, a variety of devices (ventilator, infant flow SiPAP or bubble) and interfaces (nasal prongs, nasal mask, nasopharyngeal tubes, nasal cannula) are used [11, 26]. There is no clear consensus on the level of CPAP to be applied as well as on how to wean and discontinue CPAP therapy. For instance, cycling off CPAP and transitioning from CPAP to high-flow nasal cannula (HFNC) therapy are common non-evidence-based practices.

Nasal intermittent positive pressure ventilation (NIPPV) —This has also gained popularity, with rates of use varying from 18 to 88% in different parts of the world [25–28]. It is most commonly applied as a rescue mode for infants who fail CPAP, to prevent intubation in infants with RDS or immediately after extubation. This variability in usage mainly stems from conflicting evidence on its effectiveness as well as limited understanding of its mechanisms of action, clinical indications and optimal means of delivering the pressures. Similar to CPAP, units may have at their disposal up to five different devices and interfaces for delivering NIPPV [26–28]. Synchronized NIPPV is still used by some units, but for the majority it is no longer commercially available [27, 28]. This is particularly important because the only studies demonstrating physiological and clinical benefits have used synchronized NIPPV [28].Furthermore, there is no consensus on what constitutes best settings (peak inflation pressure, PEEP and rate) and how to optimally wean NIPPV.

High-flow nasal cannula—Well before any clinical trials had established its safety and effectiveness, high-flow nasal cannula (HFNC) had been widely used across units. Surveys revealed that between 50 and 77% of units were using it [25, 29, 30]. The most common indication was in the immediate post-extubation period. In two surveys, 33% of extremely preterm infants (≤28 weeks) and 12% of infants with birth weight ≤1kg were extubated directly to HFNC, respectively [23, 30]. This is particularly concerning, given the lack of evidence for infants below 26 weeks and experts cautioning against its routine use in this population [31]. Another popular application for HFNC is as an alternative to CPAP or as a weaning step between CPAP and no respiratory support. However, no evidence currently exists to support any of those practices [32]. With regard to the actual delivery of HFNC, current evidence (from the literature and manufacturers) recommends using no more than 8 L of flow and a nasal cannula that allow some degree of leakage around the nares (around 50%). In spite of this, there is wide variability in HFNC delivery; one survey reported that as many as 15% use maximal flows greater than 8 L, over half of the respondents apply nasal cannula that exactly fits the nostrils and 23% apply measures to keep the mouth closed [29]. All these actions have the potential to deliver unreliable and dangerously high levels of pressure.

Other modes of noninvasive ventilation—More novel noninvasive modes have recently made their way into clinical practice despite the lack of evidence to support their use. Two such examples include noninvasive HFOV and noninvasive NAVA. A recent European survey reported that 17% were using noninvasive HFOV for diverse indications, mainly for CPAP failure or as primary therapy. There were significant variations in the types of equipment, interfaces and settings used for its delivery, with little information about its safety profile [33]. Similarly, noninvasive NAVA is increasingly applied in many NICUs across North America using evidence mainly based from animal data, retrospective clinical studies and case series [34].

2.5. Adjuvant therapies

Caffeine—A succession of animal, pharmacological and clinical evidence over the years has led to widespread caffeine use in neonates. The most influential publication of all was the large, multicenter Caffeine for Apnea of Prematurity (CAP) trial, which showed that caffeine significantly reduced incidence of bronchopulmonary dysplasia and cerebral palsy in preterm infants [35, 36]. Nonetheless, in the real world, caffeine practices continue to be highly variable and not always reflective of current evidence. For example, two recent surveys that reported 54 and 77% of units ensured that extremely preterm infants were loaded with caffeine prior to extubation [14, 23]. This is contrary to recommendations advocating for caffeine use in order to improve chances of successful extubations in preterm infants [37]. As another example, the use of prophylactic caffeine for the prevention of apnea has been heavily debated. The latest Cochrane review in 2010 [38] did not support routine use of prophylactic caffeine, but a series of recent retrospective studies have shown that early administration of caffeine (in the first 48 h of life) significantly reduced length of MV and improved short-term respiratory outcomes in preterm infants [39, 40]. As a result, the off-label use of prophylactic caffeine has risen from 22% (at the time of the CAP trial) to 60–75% [39, 41, 42]. The first dose is given anytime between days 1 to 25 of life and for a duration ranging from 2 to 119 days [42]. There are also noticeable differences in practices related to monitoring and discontinuation of caffeine. Ten percent of units still routinely measure caffeine levels [41]. The timing of caffeine cessation often depends on the unit's prespecified gestational age cutoff (anywhere from 32 weeks to greater than 35 weeks). A significant proportion of units also discontinue caffeine once the infant has become apnea-free for 5–7 days (81%), ≤4 days (11%) or ≥8 days (8%) [41].

Surfactant—The introduction of surfactant is probably one of the most important and life-saving discoveries in the history of neonatology. It improved survival and reduced important morbidities associated with MV, especially for the extremely preterm population. However, the role of surfactant in everyday practice has markedly evolved over time. Originally, surfactant was mainly recommended as prophylaxis for all extremely preterm infants and was preferably administered in the first 2 hours of life [43]. Nowadays, clinicians are trying to avoid MV all together and are therefore looking for alternative ways to administer it using less invasive routes [44]. As such, use of prophylactic surfactant varies anywhere between 0 and 90% [10, 11, 14, 25, 45]. Most units use the intubation-surfactant-extubation method, but other strategies are increasingly tried [46]. When surfactant is provided as rescue therapy, clinicians use different clinical indications (e.g., FiO_2 thresholds), number of doses and methods of administration (e.g. infant's position, rate of infusion, pressures and lung recruitment maneuvers used pre- and post-administration) [14, 45, 46].

Inhaled nitric oxide—The use of iNO for persistent pulmonary hypertension and acute hypoxic respiratory failure has been comprehensively studied in late preterm and term infants. In spite of this, there exists wide practice variations related to iNO administration in this population. Clinicians assess illness severity in a variety of ways (e.g., oxygenation index, pre-post ductal saturation difference, O_2 requirements and echocardiographic findings) and have different thresholds or indications to start iNO and use variable starting doses (5–20 ppm) and maximal doses (20–40 ppm) [47, 48]. Moreover, there is no standard approach for monitoring and weaning iNO (blood gases, oxygenation index, oxygen saturation and/or O_2 needs), especially in patients who are non-responders to the therapy. The most striking observation of all is the rising off-label use of iNO in preterm infants less than 34 weeks gestation, despite firm position statements and consensus guidelines recommending against it. In fact, a number of surveys and large epidemiological studies have documented wide regional and inter-hospital variations in iNO use, indications, age of initiation, dosage and duration of therapy for this group [48–50]. This raises great concern, especially when iNO is associated with staggering health costs and has not been demonstrated to improve short- or long-term outcomes in this population, with potential to cause harm in the subset of extremely preterm infants less than 1000 g [51].

3. The impact of respiratory care practice variability

For the many reasons explained in the first session of this chapter, variability in respiratory care practices is extremely prevalent. The NICU is a fast-paced environment where decisions are often made on the go and clinicians do not always have the time or sufficient knowledge to make the most informed decisions. In addition, units are often restrained in their ability to adopt a certain practice by its cost, ease of use or resource requirements (space, personnel, etc.). Most importantly though, despite the abundant existing literature, the evidence to justify most respiratory care practices is often limited or conflicting, leading clinicians to interpret study results in various ways, or shape their practices according to different background experiences and personal beliefs.

There are many implications of practice variability on patient outcomes (**Box 1**). In cases where high-grade evidence exists to guide respiratory care practices, it is easy to perceive how deviations (e.g., evidence-based therapies are introduced too late, too soon or are misused for certain populations and conditions) can negatively affect patients. But, even in cases where the evidence is unclear, the mere presence of variability has been linked to marked differences in pulmonary morbidities across NICUs. For example, rates of extubation failure range from 20 to 70% in preterm infants [52, 53]; this means that units with low extubation failure rates may perhaps be exposing infants to prolonged periods of MV while units with high failure rates may be disconnecting infants from the ventilator too soon. Both prolonged MV and the need for reintubation have been associated with serious, preventable morbidities [54, 55]. In a similar way, rates of unplanned extubation vary between 1 and 80% depending on unit MV practices and ETT fixation methods [56]. These accidental extubations also expose infants to unnecessary complications, including hemodynamic instability, need for reintubation and prolonged MV [56]. Moreover, several benchmarking studies have demonstrated important variations in the incidence of BPD across centers, which persist even after adjusting for variables known to affect this outcome [57, 58]. Authors of these studies have suggested that differences in clinical practice may actually be affecting this clustering effect. Similar observations have been made for non-respiratory related outcomes, including survival and neonatal sepsis [59–61].

Box 1.
Impact of respiratory care practice variability.

On patients

- Potential for using non-evidence-based practices
- Potential for increased errors and morbidities
- Unpredictable management
- Lack of continuity
- Parental distress

In workplace

- Increased costs
- Increased resources
- Confusion of health care team
- Inconsistent learning environment for trainees
- Reduced potential for quality control initiatives

Practice variability has potentially negative consequences that go even beyond patient outcomes (**Box 1**). It is not uncommon for a single patient to be exposed to several ventilation modes or therapies throughout hospitalization, or for a family to receive conflicting opinions regarding their child's respiratory management. This could be a great source of anxiety for the parents and may weaken their alliance with the health care team. Besides, this could create a lot of confusion among nurses, respiratory therapists and trainees, leading to lesser opportunities for productive teaching or learning. Finally, with little continuity or predictability of management, it becomes quasi impossible to effectively audit respiratory care practices or perform any quality control studies in the unit.

4. The role of respiratory care protocols in neonates

One way of harmonizing practices is through the use of respiratory care protocols. Protocols are a set of guidelines or rules to follow for a prespecified population with a prespecified condition. They have been extensively studied in critically ill adult and pediatric patients, namely for sepsis, sedation, hyperglycemia and MV. In these patients, MV protocols have consistently been demonstrated to improve outcomes by reducing costs, decreasing MV duration and shortening length of stay [62, 63]. They also have been shown to reduce rates of extubation failure as well as unplanned extubations [64, 65]. As such, MV protocols have been considered standard of care and have been developed and implemented by over two-thirds of adult ICUs [66, 67].

In contrast, the evidence for using respiratory care protocols in neonates is still limited. Studies are small, single center and retrospective or observational in nature. In one Canadian study, the implementation of a respiratory therapist-driven MV protocol for premature infants with birth weight <1250 g resulted in earlier extubation, greater number of successful extubations and shorter duration of MV [68]. In another study, the implementation of a standardized SBT protocol for extubation of extremely preterm infants resulted in faster weaning times with no impact on extubation failure rates [69]. In a further study, the implementation of a nurse-driven comfort protocol in ventilated preterm infants significantly reduced the amount of morphine used which translated in fewer days on MV and a shorter course of hospitalization [70]. Lastly, the use of a standardized surfactant protocol allowed clinicians to audit their practice and identify strategies to reduce adverse events associated with surfactant administration [71]. The results of this quality control initiative led to later modifications of the surfactant protocol, which has recently been published [72].

Despite the lack of strong evidence, it is interesting to observe that many units have already developed and implemented respiratory care protocols. In a recent Canadian survey, we showed that 38% of NICUs had at least one MV protocol, while 29% had a protocol for NIV [16]. In another international survey, 36% of units reported having a guideline or written protocol for ventilator weaning [23]. Protocols for CPAP and NIPPV are available in approximately 20% of units [16, 27, 28], while guidelines for HFNC are present in 25–50% of units [16, 29, 30].

The most striking trend is the increasing use of iNO protocols in practice. With the rising costs of iNO treatment, there have been many incentives from clinical managers and hospital administrators to audit iNO practices within their respective units. As a result, it is no surprise that almost two-thirds of units have developed and implemented iNO protocols [16]. To our knowledge, there have been no studies directly evaluating the impact of implementing iNO protocols in neonates, but there is some evidence from the pediatric literature that iNO protocols reduce practice variability, decrease iNO usage and thus lower costs without affecting mortality [73, 74]. As such, several local, national and international committees have published evidence-based guidelines to assist NICUs in developing their own institutional protocol.

Finally, there is a rising body of evidence recommending the development and implementation of clinical protocols for other specific neonatal practices or conditions. Some of these include pain control, sedation, feeding and delivery room management of extremely preterm infants (i.e., the golden hour) [75–77]. But the area in which protocols have been most well studied remains the respiratory management of neonates with congenital diaphragmatic hernia (CDH). In this population, implementation of a standardized, evidence-based protocol for respiratory care (e.g., using gentle ventilatory approaches, and permissive hypercapnia) has reliably led to lesser practice variations, improved survival and decreased morbidities [78–80].

5. Development and implementation of respiratory care protocols in the NICU

From the above sections, there is no doubt that respiratory care protocols confer many benefits. But, under some circumstances, they may also have some disadvantages (**Box 2**). Developing and implementing a respiratory care protocol is not an easy task. It requires mobilization of many collaborators, careful scrutiny of a large body of evidence and ongoing monitoring to ensure adequate application of the protocol in practice. This section will outline the key principles for effectively developing and implementing respiratory care protocols in clinical practice (also summarized in **Box 3**).

Box 2.

Pros and cons of respiratory care protocols.

Pros

- Reduces unnecessary variability in care
- Quick adoption of new information at the bedside
- Educational aids for trainees and allied health care team
- Improves communication
- Decreases costs
- Decreases errors
- Improves patient safety

Cons

- Inappropriately used for certain patients or conditions
- Oversimplified or too prescriptive
- Designed around low-quality evidence
- Potential loss of individualization of care
- Potential to be outdated if not kept current

Box 3.

General principles for effectively developing and implementing respiratory care protocols.

http://dx.doi.org/10.5772/63556

Preconception

- Obtain support from all team members

- Form a multidisciplinary working group

- Take into account that developing and implementing protocols require ample time, organization and resources

Development

- Easy to use

- Patient and disease specific

- Not too prescriptive

- Does not replace clinical judgment

Implementation

- Readily available

- Regular educational sessions

- Regular monitoring of adherence and compliance

- Periodical revision to accommodate for new evidence or clinical practice patterns

---

5.1. Preconception

Well before any protocol is drafted, it is important to take the time to get buy-in from all members of the team who will eventually be using the protocol. This includes nurses, nurse practitioners, respiratory therapists, neonatologists and their respective professional leadership. Many providers are often unaware of the negative impacts of variability on health care outcomes. Others may feel skeptical about the benefits of protocols, potentially fearing that it will take away from their ability to individualize patient care. Thus, it is of utmost importance to provide a clear rationale for using a certain protocol in the unit. Showing unit-specific data that highlight practice variations and compare outcomes with other centers may be a useful step to further justify the need for a protocol. Thus, by involving all stakeholders as early as the preconception phase, all team members will feel included and invested in the realization of the project. This will further aid in improving later rates of adherence and compliance to the protocol.

Once buy-in is obtained, the next crucial step is to create a working group that will be in charge of preparing the protocol. A member from each discipline involved in providing respiratory care (e.g., neonatologist, respiratory therapist, nurse, pharmacist and respirologist) should be encouraged to participate in this group. By using such approach, all key disciplines are represented and given the opportunity to share their perspectives. This multidisciplinary endeavor should lead to a stronger, more comprehensive and especially more inclusive protocol.

5.2. Preparation of the protocol

The development of a sound protocol depends heavily on the accuracy of its content. If a protocol is based on outdated or low quality evidence, it may actually lead to undesirable or even harmful effects. For that reason, it is essential to perform a thorough review looking for the best available evidence in the literature. Ideally, protocols should be based on results from randomized controlled trials, systematic reviews and meta-analysis. In the absence of such high-quality evidence, other studies should be carefully scrutinized with a critical mind. Additional information should be sought out from expert opinion or from other units who already have had some experience with that specific protocol. Furthermore, epidemiological databases can be a useful resource to identify centers that have better outcomes in a certain aspect of respiratory care and collaborate with them in order to identify potentially better practices responsible for these positive outcomes.

With regard to the information contained in the protocol, it should preferably be patient specific, disease specific and easy to follow. A protocol that is too flexible or unclear may lead to variable interpretations and misuses. In contrast, a protocol that is too rigid, detailed or overly specific may become inapplicable for most patients. Thus, careful attention should be placed on developing a protocol that englobes most targeted patients but that also leaves some room for individualized decision making.

5.3. Implementation and monitoring

Once the protocol is completed and approved by the necessary regulatory authorities, a number of steps need to be undertaken in order to ensure its adequate implementation. First, the protocol needs to be made readily available to all health care providers who will use it. Different channels can be used to disseminate the protocol, including the hospital intranet, monthly newsletters, posters in the unit, printed copies at the bedside and small laminated cards for staff to carry. Second, the protocol should be formally presented at educational sessions, in-services and special rounds with the aim to raise awareness, answer people's questions and clarify their concerns.

Following implementation, an effort should be made to monitor adherence to the protocol in an ongoing manner. In the absence of monitoring, it is not uncommon for protocol compliance rates to decrease with time. Thus, it is important to regularly monitor protocol usage in the unit in order to identify any major issues and promptly correct them. Regular refresher sessions may also be useful to reinforce the protocol. Finally, it is plausible that with time, new evidence-based recommendations will be made available, and hence the protocol might become outdated. As such, protocols should be revised periodically and resubmitted for approval.

http://dx.doi.org/10.5772/63556

6. Conclusion

Neonatal respiratory care involves prompt lung recruitment and adequate ventilation and oxygenation during the transition period immediately after birth to management of a variety of respiratory conditions. For this, a number of different technologies and adjunctive therapies are available with lack of high-level evidence for several of them. Thus, it is not surprising that practice variability is a reality. Respiratory care protocols are an attractive tool to promote practice standardization and reduce unnecessary variations and health care-related costs. Despite the limited evidence supporting their use in neonates, a significant number of NICUs have already developed and implemented clinical protocols into practice. Overall, respiratory care protocols appear to promote evidence-based practices, discourage outdated approaches and ultimately improve patient safety.

Author details

Wissam Shalish and Guilherme Mendes Sant' Anna*

*Address all correspondence to: guilherme.santanna@mcgill.ca

Department of Pediatrics, McGill University Health Center, Montreal Children's Hospital, Montreal, Canada

References

[1] Wyckoff MH, Aziz K, Escobedo MB, et al. Part 13: Neonatal resuscitation: 2015 American Heart Association guidelines update for cardiopulmonary resuscitation and emergency cardiovascular care. *Circulation* 2015;132(18 Suppl 2):S543–60.

[2] Singh Y, Oddie S. Marked variation in delivery room management in very preterm infants. *Resuscitation* 2013;84(11):1558–61.

[3] El-Naggar W, McNamara PJ. Delivery room resuscitation of preterm infants in Canada: current practice and views of neonatologists at level III centers. *J Perinatol* 2012;32(7): 491–7.

[4] O'Donnell CP, Davis PG, Morley CJ. Use of supplementary equipment for resuscitation of newborn infants at tertiary perinatal centres in Australia and New Zealand. *Acta Paediatr* 2005;94(9):1261–5.

[5] Trevisanuto D, Satariano I, Doglioni N, et al. Delivery room management of extremely low birthweight infants shows marked geographical variations in Italy. *Acta Paediatr* 2014;103(6):605–11.

[6] Leone TA, Rich W, Finer NN. A survey of delivery room resuscitation practices in the United States. *Pediatrics* 2006;117(2):e164–75.

[7] Hosono S, Tamura M, Kunikata T, et al. Survey of delivery room resuscitation practices at tertiary perinatal centers in Japan. *Pediatr Int* 2015;57(2):258–62.

[8] Roehr CC, Grobe S, Rudiger M, et al. Delivery room management of very low birth weight infants in Germany, Austria and Switzerland – a comparison of protocols. *Eur J Med Res* 2010;15(11):493–503.

[9] Iriondo M, Thio M, Buron E, et al. A survey of neonatal resuscitation in Spain: gaps between guidelines and practice. *Acta Paediatr* 2009;98(5):786–91.

[10] Mann C, Ward C, Grubb M, et al. Marked variation in newborn resuscitation practice: a national survey in the UK. *Resuscitation* 2012;83(5):607–11.

[11] Rocha G, Saldanha J, Macedo I, et al. Respiratory support strategies for the preterm newborn – National survey 2008. *Rev Port Pneumol* 2009;15(6):1043–71.

[12] van Kaam AH, Rimensberger PC, Borensztajn D, et al. Ventilation practices in the neonatal intensive care unit: a cross-sectional study. *J Pediatr* 2010;157(5):767–71.e1-3.

[13] Sharma A, Greenough A. Survey of neonatal respiratory support strategies. *Acta Paediatr* 2007;96(8):1115–7.

[14] Dani C, Bresci C, Lista G, et al. Neonatal respiratory support strategies in the intensive care unit: an Italian survey. *Eur J Pediatr* 2013;172(3):331–6.

[15] Alander M, Peltoniemi O, Saarela T, et al. Current trends in paediatric and neonatal ventilatory care – a nationwide survey. *Acta Paediatr* 2013;102(2):123–8.

[16] Shalish W, Anna GM. The use of mechanical ventilation protocols in Canadian neonatal intensive care units. *Paediatr Child Health* 2015;20(4):e13–9.

[17] Wheeler KI, Klingenberg C, Morley CJ, et al. Volume-targeted versus pressure-limited ventilation for preterm infants: a systematic review and meta-analysis. *Neonatology* 2011;100(3):219–27.

[18] Klingenberg C, Wheeler KI, Owen LS, et al. An international survey of volume-targeted neonatal ventilation. *Arch Dis Child Fetal Neonatal Ed* 2011;96(2):F146–8.

[19] Chowdhury O, Wedderburn CJ, Lee S, et al. Respiratory support practices in infants born at term in the United Kingdom. *Eur J Pediatr* 2012;171(11):1633–8.

[20] Tan RN, Mulder EE, Lopriore E, et al. Monitoring oxygenation and gas exchange in neonatal intensive care units: current practice in the Netherlands. *Front Pediatr* 2015;3:94.

[21] Mu TS ST, Jordan CP, UyeharaCFT. Permissive hypercapnia practices among neonatologists in the United States: results of a national survey. *J Neonatal-Perinat Med* 2011;4(2):111–7.

[22] Kapasi M, Fujino Y, Kirmse M, et al. Effort and work of breathing in neonates during assisted patient-triggered ventilation. *Pediatr Crit Care Med* 2001;2(1):9–16.

[23] Al-Mandari H, Shalish W, Dempsey E, et al. International survey on periextubation practices in extremely preterm infants. *Arch Dis Child Fetal Neonatal Ed* 2015;100(5):F428–31.

[24] Davis PG, Henderson-Smart DJ. Nasal continuous positive airways pressure immediately after extubation for preventing morbidity in preterm infants. *Cochrane Database Syst Rev* 2000(3):CD000143.

[25] Gagliardi L, Tagliabue P, Bellu R, et al. Survey of neonatal respiratory support use in very preterm infants in Italy. *J Matern Fetal Neonatal Med* 2012;25(Suppl 3):1–5.

[26] Kieran EA, Walsh H, O'Donnell CP. Survey of nasal continuous positive airways pressure (NCPAP) and nasal intermittent positive pressure ventilation (NIPPV) use in Irish newborn nurseries. *Arch Dis Child Fetal Neonatal Ed* 2011;96(2):F156.

[27] Owen LS, Morley CJ, Davis PG. Neonatal nasal intermittent positive pressure ventilation: a survey of practice in England. *Arch Dis Child Fetal Neonatal Ed* 2008;93(2):F148–50.

[28] Medeiros SK, Carvalho WB, Soriano CF. Practices of use of nasal intermittent positive pressure ventilation (NIPPV) in neonatology in northeastern Brazil. *J Pediatr (Rio J)* 2012;88(1):48–53.

[29] Ojha S, Gridley E, Dorling J. Use of heated humidified high-flow nasal cannula oxygen in neonates: a UK wide survey. *Acta Paediatr* 2013;102(3):249–53.

[30] Hough JL, Shearman AD, Jardine LA, et al. Humidified high flow nasal cannulae: current practice in Australasian nurseries, a survey. *J Paediatr Child Health* 2012;48(2): 106–13.

[31] Wilkinson D, Andersen C, O'Donnell CP, et al. High flow nasal cannula for respiratory support in preterm infants. *Cochrane Database Syst Rev* 2016;2:CD006405.

[32] Farley RC, Hough JL, Jardine LA. Strategies for the discontinuation of humidified high flow nasal cannula (HHFNC) in preterm infants. *Cochrane Database Syst Rev* 2015;6:CD011079.

[33] Fischer HS, Bohlin K, Buhrer C, et al. Nasal high-frequency oscillation ventilation in neonates: a survey in five European countries. *Eur J Pediatr* 2015;174(4):465–71.

[34] Stein H, Beck J, Dunn M. Non-invasive ventilation with neurally adjusted ventilatory assist in newborns. *Semin Fetal Neonatal Med* 2016.

[35] Schmidt B, Roberts RS, Davis P, et al. Caffeine therapy for apnea of prematurity. *N Engl J Med* 2006;354(20):2112–21.

[36] Schmidt B, Roberts RS, Davis P, et al. Long-term effects of caffeine therapy for apnea of prematurity. *N Engl J Med* 2007;357(19):1893–902.

[37] Henderson-Smart DJ, Davis PG. Prophylactic methylxanthines for endotracheal extubation in preterm infants. *Cochrane Database Syst Rev* 2010(12):CD000139.

[38] Henderson-Smart DJ, De Paoli AG. Prophylactic methylxanthine for prevention of apnoea in preterm infants. *Cochrane Database Syst Rev* 2010(12):CD000432.

[39] Lodha A, Seshia M, McMillan DD, et al. Association of early caffeine administration and neonatal outcomes in very preterm neonates. *JAMA Pediatr* 2015;169(1):33–8.

[40] Dobson NR, Patel RM, Smith PB, et al. Trends in caffeine use and association between clinical outcomes and timing of therapy in very low birth weight infants. *J Pediatr* 2014;164(5):992–8.e3.

[41] Abu Jawdeh EG, O'Riordan M, Limrungsikul A, et al. Methylxanthine use for apnea of prematurity among an international cohort of neonatologists. *J Neonatal Perinatal Med* 2013;6(3):251–6.

[42] Lista G, Fabbri L, Polackova R, et al. The real-world routine use of caffeine citrate in preterm infants: a European postauthorization safety study. *Neonatology* 2016;109(3): 221–7.

[43] Bahadue FL, Soll R. Early versus delayed selective surfactant treatment for neonatal respiratory distress syndrome. *Cochrane Database Syst Rev* 2012;11:CD001456.

[44] Gopel W, Kribs A, Hartel C, et al. Less invasive surfactant administration is associated with improved pulmonary outcomes in spontaneously breathing preterm infants. *Acta Paediatr* 2015;104(3):241–6.

[45] Horbar JD, Carpenter JH, Buzas J, et al. Timing of initial surfactant treatment for infants 23 to 29 weeks' gestation: is routine practice evidence based? *Pediatrics* 2004;113(6): 1593–602.

[46] Borszewska-Kornacka MK, Kostuch M, Korbal P, et al. Strategies of using surfactant: results of the first Polish national survey of daily practice. *Dev Period Med* 2015;19(3 Pt 1):271–6.

[47] Shivananda S, Ahliwahlia L, Kluckow M, et al. Variation in the management of persistent pulmonary hypertension of the newborn: a survey of physicians in Canada, Australia, and New Zealand. *Am J Perinatol* 2012;29(7):519–26.

[48] Sasi A, Sehgal A. Use of inhaled nitric oxide in preterm infants: a regional survey of practices. *Heart Lung* 2014;43(4):347–50.

[49] Ellsworth MA, Harris MN, Carey WA, et al. Off-label use of inhaled nitric oxide after release of NIH consensus statement. *Pediatrics* 2015;135(4):643–8.

http://dx.doi.org/10.5772/63556

[50] Stenger MR, Slaughter JL, Kelleher K, et al. Hospital variation in nitric oxide use for premature infants. *Pediatrics* 2012;129(4):e945–51.

[51] Barrington KJ, Finer N. Inhaled nitric oxide for respiratory failure in preterm infants. *Cochrane Database Syst Rev* 2010(12):CD000509.

[52] Hermeto F, Martins BM, Ramos JR, et al. Incidence and main risk factors associated with extubation failure in newborns with birth weight < 1,250 grams. *J Pediatr (Rio J)* 2009;85(5):397–402.

[53] Berger J, Mehta P, Bucholz E, et al. Impact of early extubation and reintubation on the incidence of bronchopulmonary dysplasia in neonates. *Am J Perinatol* 2014;31(12):1063–72.

[54] Walsh MC, Morris BH, Wrage LA, et al. Extremely low birthweight neonates with protracted ventilation: mortality and 18-month neurodevelopmental outcomes. *J Pediatr* 2005;146(6):798–804.

[55] Manley BJ, Doyle LW, Owen LS, et al. Extubating extremely preterm infants: predictors of success and outcomes following failure. *J Pediatr* 2016.

[56] Silva PS, Reis ME, Aguiar VE, et al. Unplanned extubation in the neonatal ICU: a systematic review, critical appraisal, and evidence-based recommendations. *Respir Care* 2013;58(7):1237–45.

[57] Lapcharoensap W, Gage SC, Kan P, et al. Hospital variation and risk factors for bronchopulmonary dysplasia in a population-based cohort. *JAMA Pediatr* 2015;169(2):e143676.

[58] Ambalavanan N, Walsh M, Bobashev G, et al. Intercenter differences in bronchopulmonary dysplasia or death among very low birth weight infants. *Pediatrics* 2011;127(1):e106–16.

[59] Alleman BW, Bell EF, Li L, et al. Individual and center-level factors affecting mortality among extremely low birth weight infants. *Pediatrics* 2013;132(1):e175–84.

[60] Lee SK, McMillan DD, Ohlsson A, et al. Variations in practice and outcomes in the Canadian NICU network: 1996–1997. *Pediatrics* 2000;106(5):1070–9.

[61] Rysavy MA, Li L, Bell EF, et al. Between-hospital variation in treatment and outcomes in extremely preterm infants. *N Engl J Med* 2015;372(19):1801–11.

[62] Blackwood B, Burns KE, Cardwell CR, et al. Protocolized versus non-protocolized weaning for reducing the duration of mechanical ventilation in critically ill adult patients. *Cochrane Database Syst Rev* 2014;11:CD006904.

[63] Blackwood B, Murray M, Chisakuta A, et al. Protocolized versus non-protocolized weaning for reducing the duration of invasive mechanical ventilation in critically ill paediatric patients. *Cochrane Database Syst Rev* 2013;7:CD009082.

[64] Bankhead S, Chong K, Kamai S. Preventing extubation failures in a pediatric intensive care unit. *Nurs Clin North Am* 2014;49(3):321–8.

[65] Jarachovic M, Mason M, Kerber K, et al. The role of standardized protocols in unplanned extubations in a medical intensive care unit. *Am J Crit Care* 2011;20(4):304–11; quiz 12.

[66] Ellis SM, Dainty KN, Munro G, et al. Use of mechanical ventilation protocols in intensive care units: a survey of current practice. *J Crit Care* 2012;27(6):556–63.

[67] MacIntyre NR, Cook DJ, Ely EW, Jr., et al. Evidence-based guidelines for weaning and discontinuing ventilatory support: a collective task force facilitated by the American College of Chest Physicians; the American Association for Respiratory Care; and the American College of Critical Care Medicine. *Chest* 2001;120(6 Suppl):375S–95S.

[68] Hermeto F, Bottino MN, Vaillancourt K, et al. Implementation of a respiratory therapist-driven protocol for neonatal ventilation: impact on the premature population. *Pediatrics* 2009;123(5):e907–16.

[69] Kamlin CO, Davis PG, Argus B, et al. A trial of spontaneous breathing to determine the readiness for extubation in very low birth weight infants: a prospective evaluation. *Arch Dis Child Fetal Neonatal Ed* 2008;93(4):F305–6.

[70] Fleishman R, Zhou C, Gleason C, et al. Standardizing morphine use for ventilated preterm neonates with a nursing-driven comfort protocol. *J Perinatol* 2015;35(1):46–51.

[71] Tarawneh A, Kaczmarek J, Bottino MN, et al. Severe airway obstruction during surfactant administration using a standardized protocol: a prospective, observational study. *J Perinatol* 2012;32(4):270–5.

[72] Nouraeyan N, Lambrinakos-Raymond A, Leone M, et al. Surfactant administration in neonates: a review of delivery methods. *Can J Respir Ther* 2014;50(3):91–5.

[73] Simsic JM, Harrison S, Evans L, et al. Reducing variation in the use of inhaled nitric oxide. *Pediatrics* 2014;133(6):e1753–8.

[74] Todd Tzanetos DR, Housley JJ, Barr FE, et al. Implementation of an inhaled nitric oxide protocol decreases direct cost associated with its use. *Respir Care* 2015;60(5):644–50.

[75] Deindl P, Unterasinger L, Kappler G, et al. Successful implementation of a neonatal pain and sedation protocol at 2 NICUs. *Pediatrics* 2013;132(1):e211–8.

[76] Kish MZ. Improving preterm infant outcomes: implementing an evidence-based oral feeding advancement protocol in the neonatal intensive care unit. *Adv Neonatal Care* 2014;14(5):346–53.

[77] Reuter S, Messier S, Steven D. The neonatal Golden Hour – intervention to improve quality of care of the extremely low birth weight infant. *S D Med* 2014;67(10):397–403, 5.

http://dx.doi.org/10.5772/63556

[78] Tracy ET, Mears SE, Smith PB, et al. Protocolized approach to the management of congenital diaphragmatic hernia: benefits of reducing variability in care. *J Pediatr Surg* 2010;45(6):1343–8.

[79] Antonoff MB, Hustead VA, Groth SS, et al. Protocolized management of infants with congenital diaphragmatic hernia: effect on survival. *J Pediatr Surg* 2011;46(1):39–46.

[80] Kimura O, Furukawa T, Higuchi K, et al. Impact of our new protocol on the outcome of the neonates with congenital diaphragmatic hernia. *Pediatr Surg Int* 2013;29(4):335–9.

Chapter 5

The Impact of Ventilation on the Development of Brain Injury in Asphyxiated Newborns Treated with Hypothermia

Asim Al Balushi, Maria A. Lopez Laporte and
Pia Wintermark

Additional information is available at the end of the chapter

http://dx.doi.org/10.5772/63385

Abstract

Birth asphyxia and the resulting neonatal encephalopathy are a significant cause of mortality and long-term morbidity in children. Hypothermia is currently the only neuroprotective treatment to have been clinically tested in large trials to prevent the development of brain injury in some term asphyxiated newborns. Most of the asphyxiated newborns treated with hypothermia are intubated at birth as per resuscitation measures and remain on mechanical ventilation during some part of the hypothermia treatment or during the whole length of the treatment. They also may present with oxygenation problems. Very often, they present with hypocapnia that can be worsened with the use of mechanical ventilation during the first days of life. When taking care of these newborns, a few important points should be remembered about the impact of asphyxia and therapeutic hypothermia on oxygenation and ventilation. In this article, we review some of the physiopathology behind neonatal encephalopathy and the implications of brain cooling from a respiratory point of view. Strategies to optimize oxygenation and ventilation for these newborns, as well as to prevent further brain injury, are also discussed based on a current literature review.

Keywords: brain, hypocapnia, neonatal encephalopathy, persistent pulmonary hypertension, ventilation

1. Introduction

Birth asphyxia and the resulting neonatal encephalopathy are significant causes of infant morbidity and mortality. Every year, three to five newborns per 1000 live births suffer from birth asphyxia and have an increased risk to die or to develop long-term neurodevelopmental sequelae [1, 2]. The sequelae may range from mild traits such as language impairments, attention deficits, and hyperactivity to more severe traits such as cerebral palsy, global developmental delay, and epilepsy [3].

Brain injury secondary to birth asphyxia and neonatal encephalopathy is a dynamic two-step process. Initially, the asphyxial insult leads to decreased blood flow to the brain (primary lesions), and this oxygen and blood deprivation around the time of birth may cause direct neuronal cell injury and cell death (necrosis) within minutes [4]. Then, as the blood flow is restored in an injured brain, a cascade of secondary pathways is initiated within the first hours and days of life that can lead to further worsening of neuronal cell injury and cell death (apoptosis) ("reperfusion injury"). Several mechanisms have been involved in these reperfusion injuries, that is, excitotoxicity from glutamate and aspartate release, disruption of calcium homeostasis, generation of oxygen-free radicals, and inflammation [2].

In the past, asphyxiated newborns were managed with supportive care only (avoidance of hypotension, avoidance of hypoglycemia, correction of blood gas parameters, and seizure control), with the goal to maintain homeostasis to limit brain injury [5]. In recent years, a number of large trials have demonstrated the efficacy of therapeutic hypothermia for the treatment of neonatal encephalopathy [6–12]. Therapeutic hypothermia is currently the only neuroprotective treatment demonstrated to be effective for preventing the development of brain injury in some term asphyxiated newborns by preventing reperfusion injuries [8] and for decreasing the risk of death and disability [1, 13, 14]. Therapeutic hypothermia involves systemic or selective head cooling of the asphyxiated newborns to an esophageal temperature of 33.5°C. Based on animal studies, the treatment has been shown to be efficient when started within 6 hours of life and continued for 72 hours, followed by progressive rewarming [6–12]. The exact therapeutic window in humans is yet to be determined.

Despite hypothermia treatment, a significant number of asphyxiated newborns still develop brain injury, and maintenance of homeostasis within the first hours and days of life is of the utmost importance.

2. Impact of birth asphyxia on oxygenation and ventilation

Brain oxygenation occurs normally through the glycolytic pathway where glucose is converted to pyruvate. This step produces the formation of the acetyl coenzyme, which enters the Krebs cycle to generate energy in the form of adenosine triphosphate through mitochondrial oxidative phosphorylation [15]. Thus, oxygen delivery to the brain cells is critical for oxidative phosphorylation to occur and for the cell to produce energy. In contrast, excessive oxygen delivery to this powerful cellular machinery will result in the generation of oxygen-free radicals leading to hyperoxia-related brain and lung injury [16]. The delivery of oxygen to the different organs, especially the brain, requires several key steps. First, oxygen is delivered from the air to the lungs. The second step occurs in the lungs at the alveolar level where the delivered oxygen is exchanged with tissue-produced carbon dioxide; this step requires adequately functioning alveoli and pulmonary vessels around these alveoli. The third step requires an adequate circulating blood flow generated by the heart to deliver the oxygen to the tissues, but also an adequate cerebral perfusion for oxygen delivery to occur in the brain. The fourth step is the extraction of the hemoglobin-bound oxygen by the tissues and its delivery to the cells.

Birth asphyxia affects the oxygenation process through several mechanisms. At the cellular level, the asphyxial event deprives cells from oxygen, and thus, pyruvate is converted to lactate through the lactate dehydrogenase enzyme. In addition, this anaerobic condition blocks the oxidative phosphorylation in the mitochondria, which leads to energy production failure, since adenosine triphosphate production is reduced [15]. In the lungs, asphyxia increases pulmonary vascular resistance, and thus the risk of persistent pulmonary hypertension, and therefore contributes to oxygenation failure, since persistent pulmonary hypertension often leads to a right-to-left shunting of deoxygenated blood, and thus a decreased delivery of oxygen to the brain [17]. This right-to-left shunting could be either intracardiac through the patent foramen ovale or through the ductus arteriosus, or intrapulmonary shunting. Also, high pulmonary vascular resistance may impair oxygenation in the absence of shunting by causing right ventricular dysfunction. Asphyxia also has a direct negative impact on cardiac function [18], and this cardiac dysfunction may contribute to oxygenation failure, since an adequate cardiac output is important for oxygen delivery to all tissues, particularly the brain. An impairment of the oxygen process has the potential to worsen brain injury in asphyxiated newborns.

Birth asphyxia leads to metabolic acidosis, mainly because the cells switch to an anaerobic metabolism as oxygen gets depleted, which leads to lactate accumulation [19]. This metabolic acidosis may lead to hyperventilation, hypocapnia, and the development of a respiratory alkalosis. Hypocapnia has been shown to exacerbate brain injury and lead to negative outcomes. Hypocapnia alters pH, reduces cerebral blood flow (through vasoconstriction and a release of vasoactive factors), alters potassium channels, and affects calcium homeostasis, all of which contribute to further damaging the brain. Hypocapnia has been associated with periventricular leukomalacia, intraventricular hemorrhage, cerebral palsy, cognition developmental disorder, and auditory deficits [20]. Thus, it may also worsen brain injury in asphyxiated newborns.

Clinical manifestations of neonatal encephalopathy include an initially altered level of consciousness, tone and reflexes, and seizures may happen [9, 21]. Respiratory difficulties are very often associated with the initial neonatal encephalopathy [21]. Most asphyxiated newborns are intubated at birth as per resuscitation measures and remain on mechanical ventilation during some part of the hypothermia treatment or during the whole length of the treatment [22].

3. Impact of hypothermia on oxygenation and ventilation

Mild hypothermia achieves neuroprotection mainly by decreasing metabolic demand and minimizing secondary energy failure. A reduction of 2–4°C of the body temperature of asphyxiated newborns can decrease their rate of cell death, delay metabolic changes, and even delay secondary brain injury [23]. The metabolic rate decreases by 5–8% with every 1°C reduction in core temperature, which in turn reduces glucose and oxygen utilization, and therefore mitigates energy failure following the initial asphyxial event [24].

Overall, hypothermia has a direct and favorable effect on oxygenation parameters (**Table 1**). Hypothermia shifts the oxygen-dissociation curve to the left, and thus, a lower partial pressure of oxygen is needed to achieve the same level of hemoglobin saturation. This left shift prevents some of the oxygen release to the tissues, which should be considered an appropriate physiological adaptation, since hypothermia also decreases the demand for oxygen. Although hypothermia has been suspected to worsen the existing pulmonary hypertension caused by asphyxia [25], larger randomized studies of asphyxiated newborns that have tested hypothermia as a treatment did not report an increased incidence of persistent pulmonary hypertension [1, 26]. In addition, hypothermia also may have an impact on lung mechanisms [27]. Asphyxiated newborns treated with hypothermia tend to have an increased compliance and a decreased mean airway pressure, and these changes tend to reverse during the rewarming process [27], and may thus predispose the newborn to a worsening of the underlying persistent pulmonary hypertension during that phase of treatment [27]. Further impairment of persistent pulmonary hypertension, and thus of oxygenation, has the potential to worsen the brain injury of asphyxiated newborns treated with hypothermia.

Parameters	Changes during hypothermia treatment	Management Strategies
Oxygen (FiO_2 and pO_2)	Lower temperature shifts the oxygen-dissociation curve to the left. Lower pO_2 are thus needed to achieve same level of hemoglobin saturation	Avoid hyperoxia (lower PO_2 may be needed to achieve same saturation)
Mean airway pressure (MAP)	Lower temperature increases lung compliance and decreases mean airway pressure	Optimize lung recruitment and avoid overdistension (lower MAP may be needed). Carefully monitor changes in lung compliance during rewarming
Ventilatory rate	Lower temperature decreases metabolic rate, and thus CO_2 production	Avoid hyperventilation by adjusting ventilatory settings
Pulmonary pressure	Lower temperature may worsen persistent pulmonary hypertension (?)	Use O_2 and NO as needed to avoid further hypoxia. Maintain adequate systemic blood pressure. ECMO to be considered when optimized treatment fails. Avoid hyperoxia
Blood gas analysis	Lower temperature decreases pCO_2 and increases pH	"pH-stat" strategy (correction of pH and pCO_2 to the body temperature) suggested as the most cautious approach

Abbreviations: ECMO, extracorporeal membrane oxygenation; FiO_2, fraction of inspired oxygen; NO, nitric oxide; pCO_2, partial pressure of carbon dioxide; pO_2, partial pressure of oxygen.

Table 1. Ventilation in asphyxiated newborns treated with hypothermia.

http://dx.doi.org/10.5772/63385

Another important factor to take into account is the variations in oxygen utilization and demand that occur during hypothermia treatment, in particular during the first few hours of life. In a previous study on asphyxiated newborns treated with hypothermia, the regional cerebral oxygen saturation measured by near-infrared spectroscopy (NIRS) increased from day 1 to 2 of life in all newborns regardless of whether they did or did not develop brain injury. However, newborns who later develop brain injury had higher regional cerebral oxygen saturation, which may reflect either more severe neuronal injury, and thus less utilization of oxygen by dead tissues, or the phenomenon of luxury perfusion that occurs when increased brain perfusion exceeds the metabolic demand [28].

As previously mentioned, hypothermia decreases metabolic rate and therefore leads to a decrease in carbon dioxide production. With respect to an asphyxiated newborn treated with hypothermia, who is breathing spontaneously, this means that any drop in the partial pressure of carbon dioxide (by a decrease in carbon dioxide production) will correlate with decreased ventilation via chemoreceptor inhibitory input into the respiratory center, in an effort to maintain a stable partial pressure of carbon dioxide. However, regarding an asphyxiated newborn treated with hypothermia, who is intubated, a risk of hyperventilation and respiratory alkalosis exits if the ventilator parameters are not adjusted to the decreased carbon dioxide production [22]. Further worsening of the hypocapnia by hypothermia may further worsen brain injury in asphyxiated newborns treated with hypothermia.

4. Evidence for best practices for ventilation in asphyxiated newborns treated with hypothermia

Most asphyxiated newborns are intubated at birth as per resuscitation measures and remain on mechanical ventilation during some part of the hypothermia treatment or during the whole length of the treatment. Past studies have reported that the ventilatory management of asphyxiated newborns treated with hypothermia is very complex [29], since it has to take into account all the previously discussed issues. The adjustment of ventilator settings should be closely fine-tuned to optimize oxygenation and limit hypocapnia in asphyxiated newborns treated with hypothermia (**Table 1**).

Mechanical ventilation in asphyxiated newborns treated with hypothermia should aim for optimal lung recruitment and avoidance of overdistension. Optimal lung recruitment should decrease atelectasis, which may reduce the effective gas exchange area in the lungs and contribute to the hypoxic pulmonary vasoconstriction [25]. In contrast, overdistension should be avoided, since it may lead to systemic hypotension by decreasing venous return, exacerbate persistent pulmonary hypertension, worsen the oxygen delivery, and thus decrease the organs' perfusion, particularly the brain [30]. No evidence from randomized controlled trials has suggested the superiority of high-frequency oscillatory ventilation over conventional mechanical ventilation in near-term and term newborns [31]. In addition, no available studies have explored which mode is the most suitable among the different possible modes of mechanical ventilation for these newborns.

After optimal lung recruitment, optimizing oxygenation consists mainly in limiting persistent pulmonary hypertension. Wide variations in the management of persistent pulmonary hypertension persist among neonatologists, which probably reflect the lack of an evidence-based approach for the treatment of neonatal persistent pulmonary hypertension [32]. In addition, the most optimal values for oxygenation parameters for asphyxiated newborns during hypothermia treatment are currently not known and probably vary according to the day of life, as has been demonstrated by the previously discussed variations in oxygen utilization and demand that occur during hypothermia treatment. Increasing the fraction of inspired oxygen has a known pulmonary vasodilator effect and should thus improve oxygen delivery and decrease the risk of further brain injury. However, this increase in the fraction of inspired oxygen should be carefully monitored, since hyperoxia or an excessive delivery of oxygen relative to the demand may lead to a worsening of brain injury through the formation of oxygen-free radicals that could at the same time worsen pulmonary hypertension [33]. Although current evidence does not support the early use of inhaled nitric oxide in preterm infants, it has been shown to decrease the need for extracorporeal membrane oxygenation in near-term and term infants with hypoxic respiratory failure [34]. Given the potential-added beneficial effect on neuroprotection and the possible impact of persistent pulmonary hypertension on brain injury, the use of nitric oxide should be considered early in the course of treatment [35]. In addition, it is important to consider cardiopulmonary interactions and optimize blood pressure in these newborns to limit the right-to-left shunting. As a last treatment resort, extracorporeal membrane oxygenation should be considered to optimize oxygenation and has been demonstrated to be feasible for asphyxiated newborns treated with hypothermia [17]. Further studies are needed to determine the most optimal values for oxygenation parameters and the best methods to reach them with respect to asphyxiated newborns treated with hypothermia.

Limiting hypocapnia is the next important step. Several studies have highlighted the importance of preventing hypocapnia in ventilated asphyxiated newborns during hypothermia [29, 36]. It remains to be established what has the worst impact on brain perfusion—a single hypocapnic episode, cumulative hypocapnia, and/or fluctuations in the partial pressure of carbon dioxide [29]. Moreover, it may be the combination of hypocapnia with hyperoxia that could lead to more adverse outcomes [36]. Alternatively, hypercapnia also should be avoided, since it has been shown to alter cerebral blood flow by causing cerebral vasodilatation and impairing cerebral autoregulation [37]. Currently, conflicting evidence exists with respect to the efficacy of permissive hypercapnia on brain protection. Although some studies have argued that it helps to avoid ventilation-induced brain injury [20], a recent study on extremely low-birth weight infants has found no significant decrease in lung injury nor mortality in newborns managed with permissive hypercapnia [38]. Permissive hypercapnia has yet to be further studied in asphyxiated newborns receiving therapeutic hypothermia. Further studies that continuously monitor the partial pressure of carbon dioxide levels and quickly adjust the ventilator settings would be necessary to improve the ventilatory management of these newborns.

http://dx.doi.org/10.5772/63385

To monitor the changes in the partial pressure of carbon dioxide and pH during hypothermia treatment and the adjustment of ventilatory settings, two strategies are available, depending on whether the partial pressure of carbon dioxide and pH are corrected or not for temperature. The "α-stat" strategy does not correct the partial pressure of carbon dioxide and pH for body temperature; rather, it measures them at normal body temperature (37°C) as is usually done for lab measurements of blood gas parameters if not specified otherwise. Alternatively, the "pH-stat" strategy adjusts the partial pressure of carbon dioxide and pH values to the actual body temperature of the newborn. At hypothermia temperature (33.5°C), the partial pressure of carbon dioxide will decrease and pH will increase compared to normal body temperature (37°C) [22, 39], since the solubility of a gas within a liquid (such as blood) decreases with lower temperature due to physical laws. A review of 16 studies comparing the efficacy of these two strategies in managing acid-base disturbances in the context of deep hypothermic circulatory arrest have suggested that the pH-stat strategy should be preferred for the pediatric population [40–44]. Such a study has not yet been performed in asphyxiated newborns treated with cooling. In the large randomized controlled trials of therapeutic hypothermia following asphyxia [9, 10], the pH-stat strategy was used, since it was considered to be the most cautious approach for maintaining the physiologic partial pressure of carbon dioxide and pH levels. With this strategy, ventilator settings need to be decreased more aggressively.

5. Conclusions

The respiratory management of asphyxiated newborns treated with hypothermia is complex. Many factors specifically related to asphyxia and hypothermia must be considered when dealing with the ventilatory management of these newborns, so to offer them the best possible level of care. Evidence is currently lacking regarding the best practices to use to optimize oxygenation and ventilation in these newborns and prevent the development of further brain injury. Further studies should be performed to determine what is the optimal mode of ventilation and what are the most optimal values for oxygenation parameters for these newborns during hypothermia treatment. Until then, the treating team should keep a very close eye on them to maintain, as much as possible, homeostasis, and to avoid hypoxemia, hyperventilation, and hypocapnia.

Acknowledgements

We thank Mr. Wayne Ross Egers for his professional English correction of the manuscript. Pia Wintermark receives research grant funding from the FRSQ Clinical Research Scholar Career Award Junior 1, and a New Investigator Research Grant from the SickKids Foundation and the CIHR Institute of Human Development, Child and Youth Health (IHDCYH).

Conflict of interest: The authors declare no competing financial interests. The study sponsors had no involvement in the study design; the collection, analysis, and interpretation of data;

the writing of the report; or the decision to submit the paper for publication. No honorarium, grant, or other form of payment was received for the preparation of this manuscript.

Author details

Asim Al Balushi, Maria A. Lopez Laporte and Pia Wintermark*

*Address all correspondence to: pia.wintermark@bluemail.ch

Department of Pediatrics, Division of Newborn Medicine, Research Institute of the McGill University Health Centre, Montreal Children's Hospital, Montreal, Canada

References

[1] Jacobs S, Berg M, Hunt R, Tarnow-Mordi W, Inder T, Davis P. Cooling for newborns with hypoxic ischemic encephalopathy. Cochrane Database Syst Rev. 2013; 1:CD003311. doi:10.1002/14651858.CD003311.pub3.

[2] Hagberg H, David Edwads A, Groenendaal F. Perinatal brain damage: the term infant. Neurobiol Dis. 2015; pii: S0969-9961(15)30057-7. doi:10.1016/j.nbd.2015.09.011.

[3] Golubnitschaja O, Yeghiazaryan K, Cebioglu M, Morelli M, Herrera-Marschitz M. Birth asphyxia as the major complication in newborns: moving towards improved individual outcomes by prediction, targeted prevention and tailored medical care. EPMA J. 2011;2:197–210. doi:10.1007/s13167-011-0087-9.

[4] Gieron-Korthals M, Colon J. Hypoxic-ischemic encephalopathy in infants: new challenges. Fetal Pediatr Pathol. 2005;24:105–120. doi:10.1080/15227950500184958.

[5] Perlman J. Intervention strategies for neonatal hypoxic-ischemic cerebral injury. Clin Ther. 2006;28:1353–1365. doi:10.1016/j.clinthera.2006.09.005.

[6] Azzopardi DV, Strohm B, Edwards AD, Dyet L, Halliday HL, Juszczak E, Kapellou O, Levene M, Marlow N, Porter E, Thoresen M, Whitelaw A, Brocklehurst P; TOBY Study Group. Moderate hypothermia to treat perinatal asphyxial encephalopathy. N Engl J Med. 2009;361:1349–1358. doi:10.1056/NEJMoa0900854.

[7] Azzopardi D, Strohm B, Marlow N, Brocklehurst P, Deierl A, Eddama O, Goodwin J, Halliday H, Juszczak E, Kapellou O, Levene M, Linsell L, Omar O, Thoresen M, Tusor N, Whitelaw A, Edwards D; TOBY Study Group. Effects of hypothermia for perinatal asphyxia on childhood outcomes. N Engl J Med. 2014;371:140–149. doi:10.1056/NEJMoa1315788.

[8] Davidson J, Wassink G, van de Heuij L, Bennet L, Gunn A. Therapeutic hypothermia for neonatal hypoxic-ischemic encephalopathy—where to from here? Front Neurol. 2015;6:198. doi:10.3389/fneur.2015.00198.

[9] Gluckman PD, Wyatt JS, Azzopardi D, Ballard R, Edwards AD, Ferriero DM, Polin RA, Robertson CM, Thoresen M, Whitelaw A, Gunn AJ. Selective head cooling with mild systemic hypothermia after neonatal encephalopathy: multicentre randomised trial. Lancet. 2005;365:663–670. doi:10.1016/S0140-6736(05)17946-X.

[10] Shankaran S, Laptook A, Ehrenkranz R, Tyson JE, McDonald SA, Donovan EF, Fanaroff AA, Poole WK, Wright LL, Higgins RD, Finer NN, Carlo WA, Duara S, Oh W, Cotten CM, Stevenson DK, Stoll BJ, Lemons JA, Guillet R, Jobe AH; National Institute of Child Health and Human Development Neonatal Research Network. Whole-body hypothermia for neonates with hypoxic–ischemic encephalopathy. N Engl J Med. 2005;353:1574–1584. doi:10.1056/NEJMcps050929.

[11] Shankaran S, Pappas A, McDonald SA, Vohr BR, Hintz SR, Yolton K, Gustafson KE, Leach TM, Green C, Bara R, Petrie Huitema CM, Ehrenkranz RA, Tyson JE, Das A, Hammond J, Peralta-Carcelen M, Evans PW, Heyne RJ, Wilson-Costello DE, Vaucher YE, Bauer CR, Dusick AM, Adams-Chapman I, Goldstein RF, Guillet R, Papile LA, Higgins RD; Eunice Kennedy Shriver NICHD Neonatal Research Network. Childhood outcomes after hypothermia for neonatal encephalopathy. N Engl J Med. 2012;366:2085–2092. doi:10.1056/NEJMoa1112066.

[12] Simbruner G, Mittal RA, Rohlmann F, Muche R; neo.nEURO.network Trial Participants. Systemic hypothermia after neonatal encephalopathy: outcomes of neo.nEURO.network RCT. Pediatrics. 2010;126:e771–e778. doi:10.1542/peds.2009–2441.

[13] Edwards A, Brocklehurst P, Gunn A, Halliday H, Juszczak E, Levene M, Strohm B, Thoresen M, Whitelaw A, Azzopardi D. Neurological outcomes at 18 months of age after moderate hypothermia for perinatal hypoxic ischaemic encephalopathy: synthesis and meta-analysis of trial data. BMJ. 2010;340:c363. doi:10.1136/bmj.c363.

[14] Shah P. Hypothermia: a systematic review and meta-analysis of clinical trials. Semin Fetal Neonatal Med. 2010;15:238–246. doi:10.1016/j.siny.2010.02.003.

[15] Vannucci RC, Brucklacher RM, Vannucci SJ. Glycolysis and perinatal hypoxic-ischemic brain damage. Dev Neurosci. 2005;27:185–190. doi:10.1159/000085991.

[16] Danilov CA, Fiskum G. Hyperoxia promotes astrocyte cell death after oxygen and glucose deprivation. Glia. 2008;56:801–808. doi:10.1002/glia.20655.

[17] Lapointe A, Barrington KJ. Pulmonary hypertension and the asphyxiated newborn. J Pediatr. 2011;158:e19–e24. doi:10.1016/j.jpeds.2010.11.008.

[18] Al Balushi A, Guibault MP, Wintermark P. Secondary increase of lactate levels in asphyxiated newborns during hypothermia treatment: a reflect of suboptimal hemodynamics (A case series). AJP Rep. 2015;6:e48–e58. doi:10.1055/s-0035-1565921.

[19] Alistair J, Bennet L. Fetal hypoxia insults and patterns of brain injury: insights from animal models. Clin Perinatol. 2009;36:579–593. doi:10.1016/j.clp.2009.06.007.

[20] Zhou W, Liu W. Hypercapnia and hypocapnia in neonates. World J Pediatr. 2008;4:192–196. doi:10.1007/s12519-008-0035-5.

[21] American college of obstetricians and Gynecologists' task force on neonatal encephalopathy. Executive summary: neonatal encephalopathy and neurologic outcome, 2nd edition. Obstet Gynecol. 2014;123:896–901. doi:10.1097/01.AOG.0000445580.65983.d2.

[22] Wintermark P. Brain cooling for asphyxiated newborns: the impact on respiratory mechanics, oxygenation and ventilation. Can J Respir Ther (CJRT). 2012;48:13–16.

[23] Selway L. Hypoxic ischemic encephalopathy and hypothermic intervention for newborns. Adv Neonatal Care. 2010;10:60–66. doi:10.1097/ANC.0b013e3181d54b30.

[24] Erecinska M, Thoresen M, Silver IA. Effects of hypothermia on energy metabolism in Mammalian central nervous system. J Cereb Blood Flow Metab. 2003;23:513–530. doi: 10.1097/01.WCB.0000066287.21705.21.

[25] Benumof JL, Wahrenbrock EA. Dependency of hypoxic pulmonary vasoconstriction on temperature. J Appl Physiol Respir Environ Exerc Physiol. 1977;42:56–58.

[26] Wood T, Thoresen M. Physiological response to hypothermia. Semin Fetal Neonatal Med. 20155;20:87–96. doi:10.1016/j.siny.2014.10.005.

[27] Dassios T, Austin T. Respiratory function parameters in ventilated newborn infants undergoing whole body hypothermia. Acta Paediatr. 2014;103:157–161. doi:10.1111/apa.12476.

[28] Peng S, Boudes E, Tan X, Saint-Martin C, Shevell M, Wintermark P. Does near-infrared spectroscopy identify asphyxiated newborns at risk of developing brain injury during hypothermia treatment? Am J Perinatol. 2015;32:555–564. doi:10.1055/s-0034-1396692.

[29] Pappas A, Shankaran S, Laptook A, Langer J, Bara R, Ehrenkranz R, Goldberg R, Das A, Higgins R, Tyson J, Walsh M; Eunice Kennedy Shriver National Institute of Child Health and Human Development Neonatal Research Network. Hypocarbia and adverse outcome in neonatal hypoxic-ischemic encephalopathy. J Pediatr. 2011;158:752–758. doi:10.1016/j.jpeds.2010.10.019.

[30] Cheifetz IM, Craid DM, Quick G, McGovern JJ, Cannon ML, Ungerleider RM, Smith PK, Meliones JN. Increasing tidal volumes and pulmonary overdistension adversely affect pulmonary vascular mechanics and cardiac output in a pediatric swine model. Crit Care Med. 1998;26:710–716.

[31] Cools F, Offringa M, Askie LM. Elective high frequency oscillatory ventilation versus conventional ventilation for acute pulmonary dysfunction in preterm infants. Cochrane Database Syst Rev. 2015;3:CD000104. doi:10.1002/14651858.CD000104.pub4.

[32] Shivananda S, Ahliwahlia L, Kluckow M, Luc J, Jankov R, McNamara P. Variation in the management of persistent pulmonary hypertension of the newborn: a survey of

physicians in Canada, Australia, and New Zealand. Am J Perinatol. 2012;29:519–526. doi:10.1055/s-0032-1310523.

[33] Konduri GG, Bakhutashvili I, Eis A, Pritchard K Jr. Oxidant stress from uncoupled nitric oxide synthase impairs vasodilation in fetal lambs with persistent pulmonary hypertension. Am J Physiol Heart Circ Physiol. 2007;292:H1812–H1820. doi:10.1152/ajpheart.00425.2006.

[34] Finer NN, Barrington KJ. Nitric oxide for respiratory failure in infants born at or near term. Cochrane Database Syst Rev. 2006;4:CD000399. doi: 10.1002/14651858.CD000399.pub2.

[35] Garry PS, Ezra M, Rowland MJ, Westbrook J, Pattinson KT. The role of the nitric oxide pathway in brain injury and its treatment—from bench to bedside. Exp Neurol. 2015;263:235–243. doi:10.1016/j.expneurol.2014.10.017.

[36] Klinger G, Beyene J, Shah P, Perlman M. Do hyperoxaemia and hypocapnia add to the risk of brain injury after intrapartum asphyxia? Arch Dis Child Fetal Neonatal Ed. 2005;90:F49–52. doi:10.1136/adc.2003.048785.

[37] Kaiser J. Neurological sequelae following mechanical ventilation. In: Berger I, Schimmel MS, Editors. Hot Topics in Neonatal Neurology. New York: Nova Science Publishers, Inc; 2008. pp. 83–107.

[38] Thome U, Genzel O, Bohnhorst B, Schmid M, Fuchs H, Rohde O, Avenarius S, Topf HG, Zimmermann A, Faas D, Timme K, Kleinlein B, Buxmann H, Schenk W, Segerer H, Teig N, Gebauer C, Hentschel R, Heckmann M, Schlösser R, Peters J, Rossi R, Rascher W, Böttger R, Seidenberg J, Hansen G, Zernickel M, Alzen G, Dreyhaupt J, Muche R, Hummler HD; PHELBI Study Group. Permissive hypercapnia in extremely low birth weight infants (PHELBI): a randomized controlled multicentre trial. Lancet Respir Med. 2015;3:534–543. doi:10.1016/S2213-2600(15)00204-0.

[39] Groenendaal F, De Vooght KM, van Bel F. Blood gas values during hypothermia in asphyxiated term neonates. Pediatrics. 2009;123:170–172. doi:10.1542/peds.2008-1955.

[40] Duebener LF, Hagino I, Sakamoto T, Mime LB, Stamm C, Zurakowski D, Schäfers HJ, Jonas RA. Effects of pH management during deep hypothermic bypass on cerebral microcirculation: alpha-stat versus pH-stat. Circulation. 2002;106:I103–I108. doi: 10.1161/01.cir.0000032916.33237.a9.

[41] du Plessis AJ, Jonas RA, Wypij D, Hickey PR, Riviello J, Wessel DL, Roth SJ, Burrows FA, Walter G, Farrell DM, Walsh AZ, Plumb CA, del Nido P, Burke RP, Castaneda AR, Mayer JE Jr, Newburger JW. Perioperative effects of alpha-stat versus pH-stat strategies for deep hypothermic cardiopulmonary bypass in infants. J Thorac Cardiovasc Surg. 1997;114:991–1000;discussion 1000–1001. doi:10.1016/S0022-5223(97)70013-8.

[42] Kurth CD, O'Rourke MM, O'Hara IB. Comparison of pH-stat and alpha-stat cardiopulmonary bypass on cerebral oxygenation and blood flow in relation to hypothermic circulatory arrest in piglets. Anesthesiology. 1998;89:110–118.

[43] Pokela M, Dahlbacka S, Biancari F, Vainionpää V, Salomäki T, Kiviluoma K, Rönkä E, Kaakinen T, Heikkinen J, Hirvonen J, Romsi P, Anttila V, Juvonen T. pH-stat versus alpha-stat perfusion strategy during experimental hypothermic circulatory arrest: a microdialysis study. Ann Thorac Surg. 2003;76:1215–1226. doi:10.1016/S0003-4975(03)00834-8

[44] Skaryak LA, Chai PJ, Kern FH, Greeley WJ, Ungerleider RM. Blood gas management and degree of cooling: effects on cerebral metabolism before and after circulatory arrest. J Thorac Cardiovasc Surg. 1995;110:1649–1657. doi:10.1016/S0022-5223(95)70026-9.

Chapter 6

Mechanical Ventilation of the Infant with Severe Bronchopulmonary Dysplasia

Edward G. Shepherd, Susan K. Lynch,
Daniel T. Malleske and Leif D. Nelin

Additional information is available at the end of the chapter

http://dx.doi.org/10.5772/63691

Abstract

Bronchopulmonary dysplasia (BPD) is the chronic lung disease of prematurity, and is the most common morbidity associated with preterm birth. Severe BPD is defined currently as a supplemental oxygen requirement at 28 days of age and a need for >30% oxygen and/or positive pressure at 36 weeks of corrected gestational age (CGA) in an infant born at <32 weeks of gestational age. The vast majority of severe BPD is characterized by high lung resistance, such that ventilation approaches must consider the relatively long time constants needed to adequately ventilate all portions of the lung to maximize ventilation-perfusion (V/Q) matching. At the same time, any ventilation strategy must take into account the vulnerable neurodevelopmental stage that characterizes the preterm infant with severe BPD. To maximize neurodevelopmental outcomes the ventilation strategy must avoid chronic use of sedation. In this chapter, we present the physiology underlying a low-rate, high-volume ventilation approach that maximizes V/Q matching, while optimizing neurodevelopment in patients with severe BPD.

Keywords: lung resistance, time constant, neurodevelopment, preterm infant

1. Introduction

Bronchopulmonary dysplasia (BPD) was first characterized by Northway and colleagues in 1967 as a chronic lung disease afflicting premature infants after neonatal intensive care unit (NICU) treatment that included administration of oxygen and mechanical ventilation [1]. Early descriptions of BPD noted profound airway inflammation, fibrosis, areas of emphysema, and a heterogeneous physiology. At that time BPD typically affected babies greater than 30 weeks of gestation at birth who weighed more than 1000 g, as few babies born earlier or smaller survived. As neonatal care has advanced, with widespread use of prenatal, antenatal, and postnatal treatments that have markedly improved survival, there has been a notable change in the epidemiology of BPD [2–4]. Such improvements in care include but are not limited to nearly universal administration of prenatal steroids to high risk infants, aggressive resuscitation practices, gentle forms of ventilation, improvements in parenteral and enteral nutrition, surfactant administration, and widespread use of nasal continuous positive airway pressure (nCPAP). The result of all these improvements in care has been marked increases in NICU survival of extremely low birth weight (ELBW) infants. While NICU survival has improved and BPD has become uncommon in infants greater than 30 weeks of gestation, rates of BPD have not changed for ELBW infants and thus the absolute number of infants diagnosed with BPD is likely increasing [5–7].

BPD is a phenotypically diverse disease with a variety of causes and consequences [8]. While previous definitions of BPD focused on a single diagnostic criteria (i.e., X-ray changes, a supplemental oxygen requirement at 28 days of age, or, more recently, a supplemental oxygen requirement at 36 weeks of corrected gestational age (CGA)) the most widely used current classifications divide BPD into mild, moderate, and severe based on the degree of support required at critical junctures. Mild BPD is defined as any supplemental oxygen requirement at 28 days of life, moderate BPD is defined as any supplemental oxygen requirement less than 0.3 FiO_2 at 36 weeks, while severe BPD is defined as a supplemental oxygen requirement with a FiO_2 greater than 0.3 and/or the need for positive pressure respiratory support at 36 weeks of CGA [9]. These changes in classification have been helpful in better defining BPD. However there remains a population of infants with the most severe forms of BPD who are not well characterized by the current classification and who represent the most difficult clinical cases typically cared for within neonatology (the severest of the severe). Such infants typically require chronic and extreme ventilator support with high peak inspiratory pressures (PIPs) and mean airway pressures (MAPs). They are often treated with high doses of neuroactive medications including narcotics, sedatives, and systemic corticosteroids. With a few notable exceptions [10], their neurodevelopmental outcomes are typically grim [11, 12]. The clinical management of patients with this degree of illness (informally known as "super-severe BPD") will be the focus of this chapter.

2. Disease progression and physiology

To understand the keys to clinical management of super-severe BPD as shown in the chest X-ray in **Figure 1**, it is critical to understand the underlying disease progression and physiology. ELBW infants are typically born at the intersection of the canalicular and saccular stages of lung embryogenesis whereas more mature infants in previous cohorts were born well after the saccular stage had commenced. This is a critical issue to understand modern, severe BPD because the stage of lung development during which lung damage occurs heavily influences both the pathological findings associated with the diagnosis and the clinical care required to manage infants with evolving BPD. Whereas older descriptions of BPD (referred to as "old BPD") typically emphasized classic progressive stages including prominent fibroproliferative changes, recent descriptions (referred to as "new BPD") have noted disruptions of distal lung growth [13, 14]. A key insight for the clinical management of the most severe forms of BPD, however, is the prominence of airway injury and dysfunction resulting from disruption of normal canalicular development.

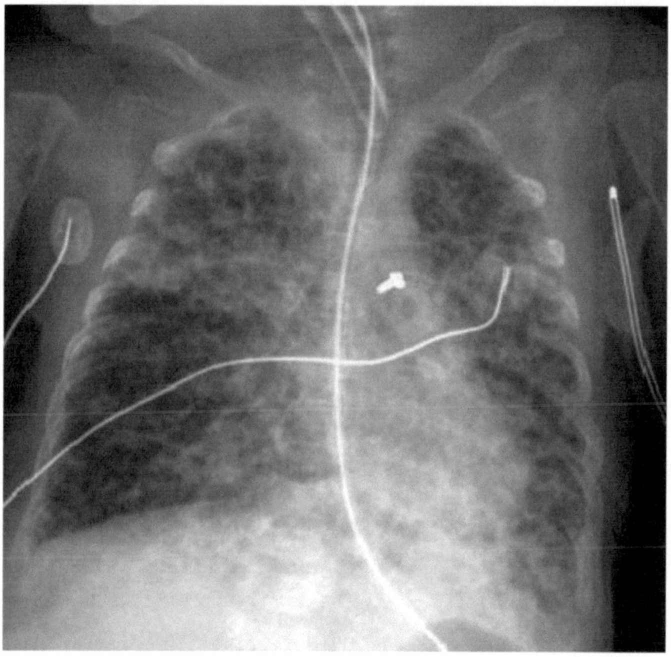

Figure 1. A typical chest X-ray for a patient with severe BPD demonstrating areas of overinflation interspersed with areas of consolidation.

Most current lung-protective strategies in neonatology are directed towards surfactant deficiency, for which extremely preterm infants are at high risk early in their NICU course [15]. Surfactant deficiency is characterized by low lung compliance (C_L, defined as change in volume for a given change in pressure or $\Delta V/\Delta P$ expressed as ml/cmH_2O) and normal lung resistance (R_L, defined as change in pressure for a given flow rate of the gas or ΔP/flow expressed as cmH_2O/ml/s). For infants in the early, acute stages of neonatal intensive care this is a very reasonable assumption, and the point of the lung protective strategy is to prevent BPD. However, this chapter discusses the mechanical ventilation of the patient with severe BPD, a relatively long time after admission to the NICU for initial respiratory care using appropriate lung protective strategies.

Let us consider how the lung fills and more importantly how the lung empties. The time needed to fill or empty is indicated by the product of C_L and R_L, termed the time constant (τ, measured in seconds). One time constant describes the time required to achieve 63% of maximal inhaled or exhaled volume, and 5 time constants are needed for 99% of maximal inhaled or exhaled volume. Since compliance is low and resistance is normal in early, acute lung disease afflicting extremely premature infants, the time required for full inflation or deflation of the lung is very short. Thus, in order to avoid overdistention and atelectasis and consequent injury, "gentle ventilation" emphasizes high-rate, low-tidal volume ventilation administered with short inspiratory times (Ti) with adequate positive end-expiratory pressure (PEEP) *via* either conventional mechanical ventilation (CMV) or high-frequency oscillatory ventilation (HFOV). Typical "lung protective" strategies suggest CMV rates of 40–60 breaths per minute (bpm), Ti of 0.2–0.3 s and tidal volumes (Vt) of 4–6 ml/kg, and for HFOV use of the minimum MAP and amplitude (ΔP) required to achieve clinical goals. Successful application of "gentle ventilation" strategies has been associated with improvements in a number of clinical outcomes including reductions in BPD, earlier extubation, and improved survival, among others. Indeed, gentle ventilation is clearly the standard of care in early, acute lung disease in extremely preterm infants.

While it may be safe to assume that early lung disease is associated with low compliance and normal resistance and can thus be adequately managed with a high-rate, low-tidal volume approach, are these assumptions valid in well-established BPD, particularly in the most severe forms? Severe BPD is often perceived to have reduced pulmonary compliance, however the predominant findings in established BPD are complex and measurement of pulmonary physiology in infants is technically difficult. The following is a summary of the current knowledge of pulmonary function in infants with the most severe forms of BPD.

3. Pulmonary function in severe BPD

While a variety of methods have been used to assess pulmonary function in infants during tidal breathing, it is critical to understand that each method has specific limitations and the results of such measurements must be understood within this context [16]. Measurements of C_L, for instance, may be variable as they are typically determined over a limited tidal volume range and depend heavily on the lung volume at which they are obtained. Further, increased airway resistance can impact measurements of C_L during tidal breathing depending on the respiratory rate. This is termed "frequency dependence" and can lead to reductions in measured compliance even in the absence of actual changes in true compliance. Other methods of assessing resistance and compliance present different problems; the single breath occlusion technique, for instance, assumes a linear, "one-compartment" model, however evidence strongly suggests that the curvilinearity of the passive expiratory flow-volume relationship in infants with severe BPD is much better described by a "two-compartment" model. Therefore, the one-compartment analysis available in ventilator software may substantially underestimate the time constant for the damaged portions of the lungs [17–19].

Despite the limitations described above, our own data combined with those of other advanced pulmonary centers describe a fairly consistent picture. In summary, infants with the most severe forms of BPD are overwhelmingly likely to have pulmonary function that is dominated by marked increases in resistance to airflow, as demonstrated by reductions in forced expira-

http://dx.doi.org/10.5772/63691

tory volume in the first 0.5 s (FEV 0.5) and in other forced expiratory flows (FEFs), with relatively normal compliance when normalized for the infant's size [20–23]. This type of pulmonary function is, in many ways, similar to that found in asthma and severe bronchiolitis and is likely the result of injury to the developing airways predominant in ELBW infants.

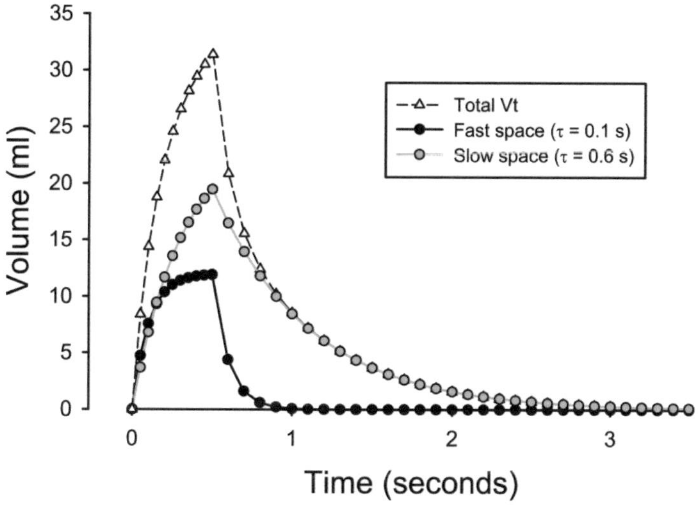

Figure 2. Volume-time curve for one breath for typical patient with severe BPD showing the fast space and the slow space. In this example, the inspiratory time is 0.5 s and the rate is 17 breaths per minute. The fast compartment (black circles) has C_L = 0.5 ml/cmH_2O, R_L = 0.2 cmH_2O/(ml/s), and τ = 0.1 s, while the slow space (gray circles) has C_L = 0.8 ml/cmH_2O, R_L = 0.75 cmH_2O/(ml/s), and τ = 0.6 s. The open triangles are the total Vt and is the sum of the volumes in the fast space and slow space. In this example the total Vt is 31.4 ml, the Vt of the fast space is 11.9 ml, and the Vt of the slow space is 19.5 ml. Clearly demonstrated is that exhalation depends entirely on the slow space as the fast space has completely emptied by 1 s, while the slow space has only completely emptied by 3.5 s, the total time for 1 breath.

The injuries to the lungs of infants with severe BPD are not regionally uniform and thus the pulmonary function of the respiratory system is heterogeneous, with some portion of the lung functioning well and other portions that are severely affected. Because of this nonuniformity, the best way to describe this heterogeneity is a "two-compartment" model with two separate and distinct sets of pulmonary mechanics [17–19]. The healthy compartment (sometimes referred to as the fast compartment) has normal or near-normal compliance and resistance, and thus a near-normal time constant. Conversely the damaged compartment (sometimes referred to as the slow compartment) is often severely injured with extremely high resistance but normal or near-normal compliance (**Figure 2**). This creates a situation in which the optimal clinical strategies necessary to achieve adequate oxygenation and ventilation will be determined by the clinician's assessment of the relative proportion of the lung that each compartment represents. Infants with relatively minimal disease, for instance, have lungs that are mostly composed of the fast compartment, while those with the most severe BPD are almost entirely slow compartment. Our own data suggest that on average 67% of the tidal volume is from the slow compartment in patients with severe BPD following bronchodilator treatment [17, 19]. This is a critical distinction as the most effective ventilatory strategy for patients with severe BPD must take into account the slow space, and the approach to ventilating the slow space is vastly different from the approach to ventilating the normal or fast space.

In addition, infants with severe BPD have significant areas of ongoing ventilation/perfusion (V/Q) mismatch and other areas of tenuous V/Q matching which lead to ongoing hypoxia and occasional "blue spells" as the tenuous area becomes intermittently poorly ventilated.

4. Physical exam, radiological, and laboratory findings in severe BPD

Physical examination findings in infants with evolving or established severe BPD are predictable but nonspecific as they represent typical findings of respiratory distress from any cause. Patients with severe BPD are typically tachypneic and will often have retractions, grunting, and nasal flaring. On auscultation wheezing and/or rales are common findings. In addition, infants with severe BPD will often be relatively hypoxic with substantial intermittent hypoxic spells that are unpredictable and often associated with movement, coughing, gagging, or bronchospasm [18]. Such infants may further appear stressed with varying degrees of hyper- or hypotonia depending on the scale of their respiratory insufficiency. On palpation, the abdomen is typically normal; however, the liver may be displaced by pulmonary hyperinflation into the abdomen and may be easily palpable.

Radiological findings in severe BPD are typically dependent on the progression of the disease. Infants in the early stages of BPD may have diffusely hazy lungs, with marked edema, and may be underinflated. As the disease evolves and becomes dominated by resistance, however, the typical chest X-ray will demonstrate hyperinflation, with relatively little direct correlation to ventilator pressures. This more likely results from breath-stacking due to prolonged expiratory time constants rather than the set ventilator pressures. Further, as the disease progresses the chest X-ray typically becomes much more heterogeneous with areas of patchy atelectasis intermixed with areas of hyperinflation (**Figure 1**).

Laboratory findings for infants with severe BPD are typically no different than for any infant with chronic respiratory insufficiency. Most notably, many such patients will have a chronic respiratory acidosis with an elevated pCO_2 and consequently an elevated serum bicarbonate. They may have a compensatory metabolic alkalosis and if blood gases are obtained they may have a substantial base excess. In addition, infants with severe BPD are at extreme risk for growth failure and osteopenia of prematurity, and thus may have associated laboratory abnormalities including elevated alkaline phosphatase, low total protein, and low albumin levels.

5. Approach to mechanical ventilation in severe BPD

There are three critical components to successfully ventilating infants with BPD. The first is that the physician must come to terms with the fact that infants with severe BPD have significantly damaged lungs that are physiologically relatively static, in other words they have

http://dx.doi.org/10.5772/63691

a chronic illness and not an acute illness. It is simply impossible for the lung function of such infants to change substantially over short periods of time (days to weeks) and it is therefore unreasonable to expect that the required respiratory support can be weaned relatively rapidly. Second, severe BPD is evolving in infants during periods of incredibly rapid neurodevelopment. Overall growth during the first few months of an extremely preterm infant's life is geometric and represents their most rapid period of growth; consequently, missed opportunities for developmental gains may be irrecoverable. Thus it is imperative that the respiratory support provided such infants be adequate to support normal interactions with their parents, family, and environment, even if requiring mechanical ventilation. Finally, the modes of ventilation used in these patients must be optimized to address the pulmonary function present in the damaged part of the lung, which likely represents the majority of the lung. Strategies that are not aimed at the diseased compartment of the lung will by definition be focused on the little remaining healthy tissue which then must compensate by absorbing the entire ventilatory load.

Since pulmonary function in infants with severe BPD is dominated by increased resistance, the expiratory time constant is very long. In infants with the most severe forms of BPD, this time constant may be as long as 0.5–0.75 s [19]. Complete exhalation, by definition, requires 5 time constants and thus may require as long as four or five seconds (5 x 0.5 = 2.5 s; 5 x 0.75 = 3.5 s). Thus, the respiratory rate must be set to allow for 5 expiratory time constants in patients with severe BPD. For if too high a respiratory rate is set on the ventilator, then there will be inadequate time for exhalation, and the subsequent breath will begin with the lung already partially inflated (breath stacking). This cycle will occur with every breath; the damaged portion of the lung will rapidly become hyperinflated, and will not be able to contribute meaningfully to overall minute ventilation (MV). Therefore the primary goal of ventilation in infants with severe BPD is to allow adequate time, in absolute terms, for complete emptying. If we take an example assuming an inspiratory time of 0.5 s and an expiratory time constant of 0.6 s, the minimum inhalation/exhalation cycle length consistent with full exhalation is 3.5 s (inhalation = 0.5 s, exhalation = 3 s), and the maximum rate that can be used on the ventilator would be 60 seconds divided by 3.5 seconds per cycle, or 17 bpm (see **Figure 2**). Any respiratory rate greater than 17, in this example, will result in breath stacking, hyperinflation, and insufficient ventilation of the bulk of the lung. This will lead to V/Q mismatch and hypoxemia which will manifest as an increasing oxygen requirement.

Carbon dioxide removal however depends on MV. MV is equal to the rate times the tidal volume (MV = rate x Vt). If the MV is 200–300 ml/kg/min, and we need to limit the set rate on the ventilator to 17 bpm to avoid hyperinflation and hypoxemia, then the only variable that we can impact is Vt. The equation can be rearranged to determine the necessary Vt as follows: Vt = MV/rate, and substituting our MV and rate gives 200–300/17 which equals a Vt of 12–18 ml necessary to provide an adequate MV at a rate of 17. A lower Vt than this will, by definition, results in inadequate MV. Furthermore, keep in mind that increasing the rate will prevent adequate emptying, leading to hyperinflation which will make the lung less compliant and thereby lead to a decrease in Vt. Essentially then, the practitioner has no alternative that is consistent with both full emptying and adequate MV other than to utilize a low-rate, high-tidal volume ventilation strategy in the patient with severe BPD.

The patient with severe BPD who is ventilated with a faster rate usually manifests air hunger demonstrated by tachypnea, retractions, and "fighting" the ventilator. These patients are often given sedatives and sometimes even paralyzed to facilitate ventilation. However in patients with severe BPD on mechanical ventilation, once a physiological slow-rate, high-tidal volume ventilation strategy is employed, the patient begins breathing more normally without air hunger. These patients usually do not require sedation and should be awake and active, such that they can interact with their environment and with therapies. Thus, this physiological ventilation strategy not only improves V/Q matching in the lung but also allows the patient to maximally benefit from neurodevelopmental therapy. Using this approach we have found that neurodevelopmental outcomes for patients with severe BPD are no longer grim, but rather are quite good [10, 24].

A small number of patients with severe BPD will not respond to this mechanical ventilation strategy. When a patient with severe BPD does not respond to slow-rate, high Vt ventilation, then the practitioner must consider rare but important causes of hypoxemia and V/Q mismatch. We recommend structure-function studies in these patients because a very small percentage of patients diagnosed with severe BPD will actually have a predominantly restrictive lung disease, and therefore will respond better to lower tidal volumes and/or PEEP. Also, there are some patients who will have tracheobronchomalacia as the predominant pathology. These patients will often benefit from relatively high PEEP to "stent" open airways on expiration. Another important cause of V/Q mismatch in this population, particularly those with severe degrees of hypoxia, is pulmonary hypertension [25]. Thus, we recommend an echocardiogram in patients who do not respond to the slow-rate, high Vt strategy with a decrease in FiO_2, or in those patients who fail to subsequently wean on the mechanical ventilator. For patients with severe BPD it is prudent to follow echocardiograms while the patients are on mechanical ventilation, since they are at high risk of developing pulmonary hypertension [26].

Once adequate MV is achieved in infants with severe BPD, it is imperative to avoid the usual acute care mentality of rapid weaning, as the underlying pathophysiology will change only with growth. In other words, once adequate MV and V/Q matching is established in the patient with severe BPD, the focus should change from weaning the ventilator to providing optimal nutrition [27]. Furthermore, the infant with severe BPD at this stage must be adequately supported at all times to allow proper neurodevelopment. In fact, attempts to wean support rapidly are highly unlikely to succeed and can impede neurodevelopmental progress putting the patient at higher risk for adverse neurodevelopmental outcomes. Our approach is to determine the most optimal ventilator settings as quickly as possible and then to delay attempts at weaning until the oxygen requirement has steadily declined to less than 40%. Optimal ventilator settings are those settings that allow for weaning of FiO_2 and allow the patient to breath comfortably without evidence of air hunger. Even when these criteria are met, it is critical to assess each infant's developmental response to therapy. If therapies are well tolerated and FiO_2 is <40% then it is reasonable to try slowly weaning the ventilator. Although we are

http://dx.doi.org/10.5772/63691

often successful extubating patients without any pressure weaning at all, if weaning is considered necessary then we recommend weaning Vt, either by decreasing PIP (for pressure-targeted ventilation) or decreasing set Vt (for volume-targeted ventilation). Each wean should be evaluated in terms of oxygen requirement and tolerance of therapies. If the wean does not result in an increase in oxygen need or a decreased tolerance of therapies then that wean was tolerated by the patient. If, on the other hand, the wean results in an increase in FiO_2 or poor tolerance of therapies then that wean was not tolerated and the ventilator should be turned up again to the previous settings. Once extubation criteria are met (**Table 1**) and the patient is successfully extubated, infants with severe BPD will often need prolonged noninvasive positive pressure via nCPAP, which should only be weaned once the infant is thriving on relatively low amounts of supplemental oxygen (25–30%). Obviously, these patients will likely need supplemental oxygen therapy for a relatively long time. Although it is rare in our practice to discharge patients home on mechanical ventilation or positive pressure, the majority of our patients are, i.e. patients are discharged home on supplemental discharged home on supplemental oxygen.

No airway anomalies
Thriving with FiO_2 ≤0.4 for at least 48 h
No recent escalation in respiratory support
Positive weight trend and good linear growth
Full enteral feeds
No surgery planned for at least 72 h
No ROP examination on day of extubation
No active infections
All needed extubation medications ordered
No recent extubation failures
Team consensus that the patient is ready

Table 1. Extubation criteria for infants with severe BPD.

6. Conclusions

Infants with severe BPD are at extreme risk for morbidity and mortality. The vast majority of these infants, however, has fairly predictable pulmonary mechanics, characterized by high resistance. Once these pulmonary mechanics are understood, it is usually possible to adequately ventilate these babies using a physiological, low-rate, high-tidal volume approach aimed at supporting ongoing neurodevelopment. It is imperative to adequately support these patients for a relatively long time to allow for lung growth and neurodevelopment. The temptation to wean these patients rapidly, as we do for acutely ill patients, must be avoided to allow for optimal outcomes.

Author details

Edward G. Shepherd*, Susan K. Lynch, Daniel T. Malleske and Leif D. Nelin

*Address all correspondence to: Edward.Shepherd@nationwidechildrens.org

Comprehensive Center for Bronchopulmonary Dysplasia, Nationwide Children's Hospital, Columbus, OH, USA and Department of Pediatrics, The Ohio State University College of Medicine, Columbus, Ohio, USA

References

[1] Northway, W.J., R.C. Rosan, and D.Y. Porter, Pulmonary disease following respirator therapy of hyaline-membrane disease. Bronchopulmonary dysplasia. N Engl J Med, 1967. 276(7): p. 357–368.

[2] Rojas, M.A., et al., Changing trends in the epidemiology and pathogenesis of neonatal chronic lung disease. J Pediatr, 1995. 126(4): p. 605–610.

[3] Bancalari, E., N. Claure, and I.R. Sosenko, Bronchopulmonary dysplasia: changes in pathogenesis, epidemiology and definition. Semin Neonatol, 2003. 8(1): p. 63–71.

[4] Kinsella, J.P., A. Greenough, and S.H. Abman, Bronchopulmonary dysplasia. Lancet, 2006. 367(9520): p. 1421–1431.

[5] Stoll, B.J., et al., Trends in care practices, morbidity, and mortality of extremely preterm neonates, 1993–2012. JAMA, 2015. 314(10): p. 1039–1051.

[6] Laughon, M., et al., Antecedents of chronic lung disease following three patterns of early respiratory disease in preterm infants. Arch Dis Child Fetal Neonatal Ed, 2011. 96(2): p. F114-F120.

[7] Latini, G., et al., Survival rate and prevalence of bronchopulmonary dysplasia in extremely low birth weight infants. Early Hum Dev, 2013. 89(Suppl 1): p. S69-S73.

[8] Lal, C.V. and N. Ambalavanan, Biomarkers, early diagnosis, and clinical predictors of bronchopulmonary dysplasia. Clin Perinatol, 2015. 42(4): p. 739–754.

[9] Ehrenkranz, R.A., et al., Validation of the National Institutes of Health consensus definition of bronchopulmonary dysplasia. Pediatrics, 2005. 116(6): p. 1353–1360.

[10] Shepherd, E.G., et al., An interdisciplinary bronchopulmonary dysplasia program is associated with improved neurodevelopmental outcomes and fewer rehospitalizations. J Perinatol, 2012. 32(1): p. 33–38.

[11] DeMauro, S.B., et al., Developmental outcomes of very preterm infants with tracheostomies. J Pediatr, 2014. 164(6): p. 1303–1310 e2.

[12] Laptook, A.R., et al., Adverse neurodevelopmental outcomes among extremely low birth weight infants with a normal head ultrasound: prevalence and antecedents. Pediatrics, 2005. 115(3): p. 673–680.

[13] Jobe, A.J., The new BPD: an arrest of lung development. Pediatr Res, 1999. 46(6): p. 641–643.

[14] Baraldi, E. and M. Filippone, Chronic lung disease after premature birth. N Engl J Med, 2007. 357(19): p. 1946–1955.

[15] Jobe, A.H., What is RDS in 2012? Early Hum Dev, 2012. 88(Suppl 2): p. S42-S44.

[16] Gappa, M., et al., Lung function tests in neonates and infants with chronic lung disease: lung and chest-wall mechanics. Pediatr Pulmonol, 2006. 41(4): p. 291–317.

[17] Jarriel, W.S., et al., A nonlinear regression analysis of nonlinear, passive-deflation flow-volume plots. Pediatr Pulmonol, 1993. 15(3): p. 175–182.

[18] Abman, S.H. and L.D. Nelin, Management of the infant with severe bronchopulmonary dysplasia, in The Newborn Lung: Neonatology Questions and Controversies, E. Bancalari, Editor. 2012, Elsevier Saunders: Philadelphia, PA. p. 407–425.

[19] Castile, R.G. and L.D. Nelin, Lung function, structure and the physiologic basis for mechanical ventilation of infants with established BPD, in Bronchopulmonary Dysplasia, S. Abman, Editor. 2010, Informa Healthcare: New York, NY. p. 328–246.

[20] Baraldi, E., et al., Pulmonary function until two years of life in infants with bronchopulmonary dysplasia. Am J Respir Crit Care Med, 1997. 155(1): p. 149–155.

[21] Gerhardt, T., et al., Serial determination of pulmonary function in infants with chronic lung disease. J Pediatr, 1987. 110(3): p. 448–456.

[22] Fakhoury, K.F., et al., Serial measurements of lung function in a cohort of young children with bronchopulmonary dysplasia. Pediatrics, 2010. 125(6): p. e1441–e1447.

[23] Thunqvist, P., et al., Lung function at 6 and 18 months after preterm birth in relation to severity of bronchopulmonary dysplasia. Pediatr Pulmonol, 2015. 50(10): p. 978–986.

[24] Trittmann, J.K., L.D. Nelin, and M.A. Klebanoff, Bronchopulmonary dysplasia and neurodevelopmental outcome in extremely preterm neonates. Eur J Pediatr, 2013. 172(9): p. 1173–1180.

[25] Mourani, P.M. and S.H. Abman, Pulmonary hypertension and vascular abnormalities in bronchopulmonary dysplasia. Clin Perinatol, 2015. 42(4): p. 839–855.

[26] Trittmann, J.K., et al., Arginase I gene single-nucleotide polymorphism is associated with decreased risk of pulmonary hypertension in bronchopulmonary dysplasia. Acta Paediatr, 2014. 103(10): p. e439–e443.

[27] Biniwale, M.A. and R.A. Ehrenkranz, The role of nutrition in the prevention and management of bronchopulmonary dysplasia. Semin Perinatol, 2006. 30(4): p. 200–208.

Chapter 7

Respiratory Distress and Management Strategies in the Newborn

Begüm Atasay, İlke Mungan Akın and Serdar Alan

Additional information is available at the end of the chapter

http://dx.doi.org/10.5772/64397

Abstract

Approximately 10% of neonates require respiratory support immediately after delivery due to transitional problems or respiratory disorders, and up to 1% of neonates are in need of resuscitation. Respiratory distress is the most frequent cause of neonatal intensive care unit (NICU) admission, and the individual management strategies should be the main task in NICUs for these infants. Regardless of the cause, if not recognized and managed in advance, respiratory distress can escalate to respiratory failure and cardiopulmonary arrest. This chapter explores the evaluation and differential diagnosis of respiratory distress in neonates and presents an update on management strategies according to the protocol of Ankara University Children's Hospital Neonatal Intensive Care Unit.

Keywords: respiratory distress, newborn, transient tachypnea, respiratory distress syndrome, neonatal pneumonia, management

1. Introduction

Approximately 10% of neonates require respiratory support immediately after delivery due to transitional problems or respiratory disorders, and up to 1% of neonates are in need of resuscitation. Respiratory distress is the most frequent cause of neonatal intensive care unit (NICU) admission, and the individual management strategies should be the main task in NICUs for these infants. Fifteen percent of term infants and twenty-nine percent of late preterm infants admitted to the NICU develop significant respiratory morbidity; this is even higher for infants born before 34 weeks' gestation.

Regardless of the cause, if not recognized and managed in advance, respiratory distress can escalate to respiratory failure and cardiopulmonary arrest. Therefore, it is imperative that any health care practitioner caring for newborn infants can readily recognize the signs and symptoms of respiratory distress, differentiate various causes, and initiate management strategies to prevent significant complications or death. [1]

2. Evaluation of the newborn infant's respiratory status

Respiratory distress is recognized as any signs of labored breathing in the neonate. Recognition of these signs and symptoms is important for both diagnosis and evaluation of the response to treatment [2].

A thorough history may guide in identifying risk factors associated with common causes of neonatal respiratory distress. Together with former and present obstetric history, gestational age, birth weight, presence of fetal distress, maternal diseases, medications, exposure to antenatal steroid, mode and duration of delivery, need for resuscitation, timing, and severity of signs and symptoms are all important for initial evaluation and decision making.

A detailed physical examination should focus beyond the lungs to identify non-pulmonary causes, such as airway obstruction, abnormalities of the chest wall, and cardiovascular or neuromuscular disease that may initially present as respiratory distress in a newborn [1]. Careful inspection and auscultation are important. Signs of increased work of breathing (WOB) [1], such as tachypnea, nasal flaring, retractions, bilateral and equal aeration of the lung and breath sounds, and the presence of cyanosis, should be evaluated. Noisy breathing may

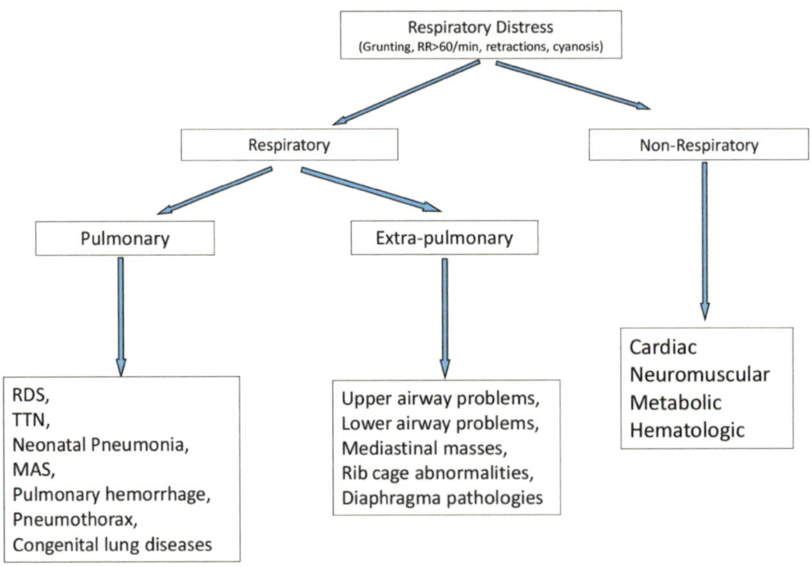

Figure 1. Etiologies of respiratory distress in the newborns.

http://dx.doi.org/10.5772/64397

indicate increased airway resistance, and the type of noise auscultation such as grunting, stridor, and wheezing may help to localize airway obstruction [1].

Non-invasive pulse oximetry is recommended by the American Heart Association (AHA) guideline for neonatal resuscitation in 2015 [3] and the American Academy of Pediatrics (AAP) to screen infants for hypoxemia, and saturation oxygen (SpO_2) values less than 85% are considered normal before 5 minutes of age [3, 4]. The partial pressure of transcutaneous CO_2 ($PtCO_2$) is considered as an accurate estimate of both arterial and venous CO_2 tension in newborn [5]. Blood pressure, heart rate follow, and frequent assessment of capillary refill time also give clues about the infants' well being.

Chest X-ray can reveal congenital malformations, and intrathoracic space-occupying lesions, such as pneumothorax, mediastinal mass, and congenital diaphragmatic hernia (CDH), can compromise lung expansion [1].

Blood gas analysis may vary according to gestational age and underlying disease of the newborns. Targeted arterial blood gas values are shown in **Table 1** [6].

Gestational age	Arterial blood gas values				
	pH	PaO_2 (mm Hg)	$PaCO_2$ (mm Hg)	HCO_3 (mEq/L)	BE
<30 weeks	7.27–7.32	45–60	45–60	19–22	±4
30–36 weeks	7.30–7.35	50–70	45–55	22–25	±3
>36 weeks	7.32–7.38	60–80	35–45	24–26	±3
Term with PPHT	7.35–7.45	80–100	30–45	24–26	±3
BPD	7.35–7.45	50–80	55–65	22–25	±3

Table 1. Range of acceptable arterial blood gas values according to gestational age. Adapted from Ref. [4].

Neonatal respiratory distress is not due to respiratory origin. Thus, after initial resuscitation and stabilization, it is important to attain a detailed history, physical examination, and radiographic and laboratory analyses to determine a more specific diagnosis and tailor an appropriate individual management as soon as possible (**Figure 1**).

Significant tachypnea without increased work of breathing (WOB) should prompt additional laboratory investigation to identify metabolic acidosis or sepsis [1].

Most of the time it may be difficult to distinguish cardiovascular diseases from pulmonary causes of respiratory distress. Most congenital heart defects present with cyanosis, tachypnea, or respiratory distress from cardiac failure. Timing of the symptoms is an important clue for most of the conditions as very few congenital heart defects present immediately after birth [1]. Cardiac pathology should be suspected especially when there is persistent cardiomegaly, abnormal pulses, or a postductal SaO_2 drop.

Regardless of the cause, it is vital to recognize symptoms and act quickly. Non-specific treatment and respiratory support started even before the specific underlying diagnosis. If the newborn cannot sustain the extra WOB to meet its respiratory needs, respiratory failure follows. This failure may manifest as impaired oxygenation (cyanosis) or ventilation (respiratory acidosis). Without prompt intervention, respiratory arrest is imminent.

3. Common diseases causing neonatal respiratory distress

3.1. Transient tachypnea of neonate

Transient tachypnea of neonate (TTN) is a benign self-limited, common respiratory disease of term and late preterm infants due to impaired clearance of lung liquid. Rapid clearance of fetal lung fluid is a key aspect of the transitional period in the delivery room [7]. Hooper et al. [8], who used phase contrast X-ray imaging to observe the rate and spatial pattern of lung aeration at birth in rabbit pups delivered by cesarean section, found the close association of residual liquid clearance from the airways with the present inspiratory activity. They detected no significant distal movement of the air/liquid interface between breaths. These findings indicate that the transpulmonary pressure generated by inspiratory effort also plays a critical role in the airway fluid clearance [8]. The clearance of fetal lung fluid mainly depends on two mechanisms: amiloride-sensitive sodium transport through epithelial sodium channels in lung and mechanical forces created during vaginal delivery. Actually, lungs of preterm infants are less responsive to this sodium reabsorption, leading to less efficient lung fluid clearance [9]. Pathophysiology of TTN and RDS is assumed to be related to the disruption of this process [7]. In our study, we suggested the possible relationship of lower cord levels of cortisol, adrenocorticotrophic hormone, and free triiodothyronine in TTN group with fetal lung fluid clearance and hormonal modulatory effect on postnatal pulmonary adaptation [10]. Thus, interruption of this process at any step such as delivery before onset of labor or delay in the first breath may result in transition problems including TTN.

Delivery following elective cesarean section (C/S) is the main risk factor for TTN. The usual mechanisms present with the onset of labor for the clearance of lung fluid in vaginal delivery are often inadequate after elective C/S, resulting in TTN [11]. Other risk factors are delivery prior to 39 weeks of gestation, precipitous delivery, fetal distress, male sex, low birth weight and macrosomia [12], multiple gestations and maternal sedation, and maternal diseases such as gestational diabetes and asthma [13].

Incidence of TTN requiring ventilation is significantly reduced to each extra week in utero decreasing from 34% at 37 weeks to 0.5% at 41 weeks of gestation [14]. In European Consensus Guidelines on the Management of Neonatal Respiratory Distress Syndrome in Preterm Infants – Update 2013 [15], antenatal steroids are also considered for women undergoing a C/S prior to labor up to term. As the long-term effects are currently unknown, at present, the best course is to avoid elective C/S prior to 39 weeks wherever possible.

The infant is usually term, near term or large, and premature, and shortly after delivery or within the first 6 hours of delivery has tachypnea. It usually presents with grunting and other mild signs of respiratory distress because lung liquid inhibits gas exchange, which persists for up to 48 hours.

Continuous pulse oximetry follow-up is needed. Blood gases often reveal some degree of mild to moderate hypoxemia. Partial CO_2 pressure is usually normal due to tachypnea but sometimes either hypocarbia or mild hypercarbia may exist resulting in mild respiratory acidosis [16].

Complete blood count (CBC) is needed for differentiation of sepsis, neonatal pneumonia, and polycythemia because CBC is normal in TTN.

Chest radiographs reveal hyperinflation, which is a hallmark of TTN. There are excess diffuse parenchymal infiltrates due to fluid in the interstitium, fluid in the interlobar fissure, and occasionally pleural effusions. Mild to moderate cardiomegaly with flattened diaphragm and prominent pulmonary vascular markings may also be present (**Figure 2a**).

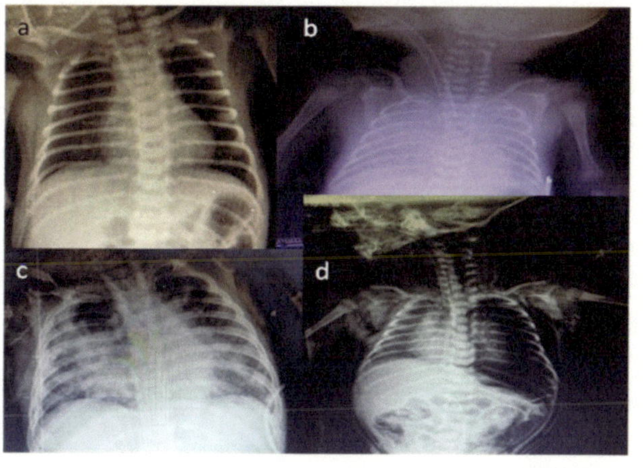

Figure 2. Chest X-ray of a newborn with (a) transient tachypnea of the newborn, (b) respiratory distress syndrome, (c) meconium aspiration syndrome, and (d) pneumothorax.

3.2. Neonatal pneumonia

Among newborns with respiratory distress, the third most likely cause after RDS (46%) and TTN (37%) is pneumonia. The incidence of pneumonia/sepsis in preterm infants with birth weight 1500–2500 g is only 0.28%, whereas in patients with birth weight <1000 g, the incidence is severalfold higher at 1.9% [17].

Respiratory infections in the newborn may be bacterial, viral, fungal, spirochetal, or protozoan in origin. Infants may acquire pneumonia transplacentally (congenital pneumonia), through infected amniotic fluid, through colonization at the time of birth, from the community or nosocomially [18]. Perinatal pneumonia is the most common form of neonatal pneumonia and is acquired at birth. Common pathogens include Group B streptococcus (GBS), gram-positive bacteria, *Streptococcus pneumonia, Staphylococcus aureus, Listeria,* and gram-negative enteric rods (e.g. *E. coli*); and viruses, such as herpes simplex virus, respiratory syncytial virus, and influenza A & B viruses; atypical organisms, such as chlamydia; and fungi [19]. Risk factors for perinatal pneumonia include prolonged rupture of membranes (PROMs), maternal infection (maternal fever or raised white cell count), and prematurity [19]. Birth weight and age of onset are both strongly associated with the mortality risk from pneumonia. Pneumonia can occur secondary to invasive mechanical ventilation but is largely confined to preterm infants who receive prolonged ventilation. Prevention of neonatal pneumonia and its complications focuses on maternal GBS screening, intrapartum antibiotic prophylaxis, and appropriate follow-up of newborns at high risk after delivery [20, 21]. On the other hand, the most important and easiest method of preventing nosocomial pneumonia is hand washing to prevent cross-infection and avoiding invasive ventilation [19–21].

Pneumonia in newborn infants is often difficult to diagnose and distinguish from other causes of respiratory distress including RDS and TTN. Infants present with increased WOB and oxygen requirement. In contrast to older infants and children, neonatal pneumonia is part of a generalized sepsis illness; thus, obtaining investigations including blood white cell counts, CRP even though they lack the necessary sensitivity and specificity to accurately diagnose pneumonia, blood, and cerebrospinal fluid cultures and initiating broad-spectrum antibiotic therapy is recommended for any symptomatic infant [19, 20]. Unlike TTN, RDS, and MAS, bacterial infection takes time to develop with respiratory consequences occurring hours to days after birth.

Chest radiography helps in the diagnosis with bilateral diffuse parenchymal infiltrates with air bronchograms or lobar consolidation suggesting in utero infection. Pleural effusions are present in two thirds of cases [22].

3.3. Respiratory distress syndrome

Respiratory distress syndrome (RDS), formerly called hyaline membrane disease, is caused by a deficiency of surfactant and is often, which strictly speaking, a histological diagnosis. The Vermont Oxford Network definition for RDS requires an arterial oxygen tension (PaO_2) <50 mmHg and central cyanosis in room air, a requirement for supplemental oxygen to maintain PaO_2 >50 mmHg, or a requirement for supplemental oxygen to maintain a pulse oximeter saturation over 85% and a characteristic chest radiographic appearance within the first 24 hours of life [23].

The EuroNeoNet figures for 2010 show an incidence of 92% at 24–25 weeks' gestation, 88% at 26–27 weeks, 76% at 28–29 weeks, and 57% at 30–31 weeks [24]. However, published data have shown that infants with a birth weight of >2500 g account for 9.9–11.5% of infants with RDS, and those with gestational age of 37 weeks' gestation account for 7.8% [12].

Pathophysiologic mechanisms include as follows:

A- Surfactant deficiency increases surface tension in alveoli, resulting in microatelectasis and widespread alveolar collapse. In the absence of surfactant, the small airspaces collapse; each expiration results in progressive atelectasis. Exudative proteinaceous material and epithelial debris, resulting from progressive cellular damage, accumulate in the airway and directly decrease total lung capacity.

B- In the presence of a weak, compliant chest wall secondary to prematurity, the large negative pressures generated to open the collapsed airways cause retraction and floppy chest wall instead of proper inflation and stability [23].

C- The presence or absence of a cardiovascular shunt through a patent ductus arteriosus (PDA) may change the presentation or course of the disease.

Decreasing gestational age is inversely related to the RDS risk. Dani et al. reported the main risk factors for RDS as gestational age, low birth weight, maternal age, elective and emergency C/S, and male sex [12]. Type II cells responsible for surfactant synthesis are sensitive to asphyxia. Their maturation can be delayed with the presence of fetal hyperinsulinemia. On the contrary, administration of antenatal corticosteroids, chronic intrauterine stress due to pregnancy-induced hypertension, intrauterine growth restriction, or twin gestation enhances their maturity [23].

Preventing premature birth will lower the incidence of RDS. Prenatal steroids decrease the risk of RDS and additionally decrease the risk of intraventricular hemorrhage and NEC [24]. Twenty-four milligrams of betamethasone therapy is recommended in all pregnancies with threatened preterm labor below 35 weeks' gestation. The optimal time period between the treatment and delivery is more than 24 hours and less than 7 days after the first dose of steroid [24]. After 14 days, benefits are diminished. A single repeat course a week after the first course reduces not only RDS and other short-term problems but also birth weight [25]. Using antibiotics in the case of preterm prelabor rupture of the membranes can delay delivery [26]. Tocolytics are mainly used to allow safe transfer to a suitable perinatology center and/or enable steroid effect [27, 28].

The clinical course of the disease varies with the presence of antenatal steroid, severity of disease, size of the infant, use of surfactant, the presence of infection, and degree of shunting of blood through PDA. With modern early management, classical definition of RDS may not be achieved, and making the diagnosis on the basis of having administered surfactant may be an overestimate [23].

Infants with RDS typically present within the first several hours of life, often immediately after delivery or in the first hours of life with marked respiratory distress and significant need of supplemental oxygen. The course of RDS is self-limited and typically improves by age 3–4 days in correlation with the aforementioned diuresis phase and as the infant begins to produce endogenous surfactant.

Blood gas sampling reveals hypoxemia with hypercarbia. Without intervention, worsening of blood gases will correlate the clinical status of the patient.

Complete blood count and blood culture should be obtained from each infant as early onset sepsis can be indistinguishable from RDS.

Chest radiography typically shows uniform reticulogranular pattern, referred to as a ground-glass appearance with peripheral air bronchograms (**Figure 2b**).

3.4. Persistent pulmonary hypertension of the neonate

Persistent pulmonary hypertension (PPHN) is a condition characterized by marked pulmonary hypertension resulting from elevated pulmonary vascular resistance (PVR) and altered pulmonary vasoreactivity, leading to right-to-left shunting of blood through intra or extrapulmonary shunts (foramen ovale or PDA) [29]. It can be either primary or secondary due to conditions leading to hypoxemia such as RDS, congenital diaphragmatic hernia (CDH), MAS, and pneumonia. Events such as perinatal stress, hemorrhage, aspiration, hypoxia, and hypoglycemia may lead to PPHN. On the other hand, PPHN may be the result of underdevelopment of the lung together with its vascular bed (e.g., CDH and hypoplastic lungs) [19, 29]. Right-to-left shunting of blood through foramen ovale or PDA due to high PVR further contributes to systemic hypoxemia and metabolic acidemia, both of which contribute to ongoing increased PVR. Ventilation perfusion mismatching is also likely to be present compounded by conditions such as MAS [19]. Risk factors can be classified as conditions related to lungs such as MAS, RDS, pneumonia, pulmonary hypoplasia, and CDH and conditions related to other systemic disorders (such as polycythemia, hypoglycemia, hypoxia, acidosis, hypocalcemia, hypothermia, and sepsis) or some of the congenital heart diseases (total anomalous venous return and hypoplastic left heart). Perinatal asphyxia, CNS disorders, and neuromuscular diseases can also result in PPHN [29]. Resuscitation and support from birth may presumably prevent or ameliorate, to some degree, PPHN when it may occur superimposed on a preexisting condition.

Pulmonary hypertension needs to be considered in any infants with respiratory distress and cyanosis. This may occur despite adequate ventilation. It is often challenging to manage and usually presents in the first few hours of life but may present later especially when secondary to the other conditions. It is also associated with significant mortality especially if associated with CDH [30]. When PPHN occurs without concurrent pulmonary disease, differentiating from cyanotic heart disease is difficult. In an infant with pulmonary disease, PPHN should be suspected as a complicating factor when there is marked hypoxemia and liability in oxygenation. These infants may have significant decrease in pulse oximetry readings with routine nursing care or minor stress [29]. The response to ventilation with 100% oxygen (hyperoxia test) can help distinguish the two conditions. In some neonates with PPHN, the PaO_2 will increase above 100 mmHg, whereas it will not increase above 45 mmHg in infants with cyanotic heart defects that have circulatory mixing [29].

Physical findings may include a prominent right ventricular impulse, a single second heart sound, and a murmur of tricuspid insufficiency. In extreme cases, there may be hepatomegaly and signs of heart failure [29].

In the presence of right-to-left shunting of blood through the PDA, a difference >10–15 mmHg of the PaO_2 is present between the preductal blood (from the right radial artery) and the postductal blood (obtained from other extremities or umbilical artery).

The chest X-ray differs according to the cardiac functions and the presence of pulmonary disease. Normal or decreased pulmonary vascularity and normal-sized heart or cardiomegaly can be observed [29].

Echocardiography is essential in distinguishing cyanotic congenital heart disease from PPHN because the latter frequently is a diagnosis of exclusion.

3.5. Meconium aspiration syndrome

Meconium is composed of lanugo, bile, vernix, pancreatic enzymes, desquamated epithelia, amniotic fluid, and mucus. Meconium is present in the gastrointestinal tract as early as 16 weeks' gestation but is not present in the lower descending colon until 34 weeks' gestation; therefore, meconium stained amnion fluid (MSAF) is seldom seen in infants younger than 37 weeks' gestation [31]. In the compromised fetus, hypoxia or acidosis may result in a peristaltic wave and relaxation of the anal sphincter, resulting in meconium passage in utero. The passage of meconium in utero results in MSAF, which may be aspirated by the fetus especially if already compromised, during gasping [19]. Any infant who is born through MSAF and develops respiratory distress after delivery, which cannot be attributed to another cause, is diagnosed as having MAS. Meconium aspiration syndrome is essentially a disease of term and post-term born infants, but an infective etiology especially from Listeria should be suspected in preterm deliveries associated with MSAF [19]. Meconium can cause mechanical obstruction of the airways leading to mismatched ventilation/perfusion. Meconium is toxic to the newborn lung, causing inflammation and epithelial injury as it migrates distally. The pH of meconium is 7.1–7.2. The acidity causes airway inflammation, chemical pneumonitis, and infection, which inhibits surfactant function and leads to inflammation and swelling, which also can block small airways with release of cytokines [1, 31]. As meconium reaches the small airways, partial obstruction occurs, which results in air trapping and hyperaeration. Thick MSAF, post-term gestational age, fetal distress, male sex, APGAR score <7 at 5 minutes, and oligohydramnios are the main risk factors. Previously, many post-term infants (>42 weeks' gestation) developed MAS. Reducing post-term deliveries has been shown to reduce the incidence of MAS [32]. In addition, advances in fetal heart rate monitoring have identified compromised fetuses, allowing for timely obstetric intervention that may help to prevent in utero aspiration of meconium. Amnioinfusion or transcervical infusion of saline into the amniotic cavity has been proposed, but best evidence does not indicate a reduced risk of moderate to severe MAS or perinatal death [33].

Endotracheal suctioning immediately after birth was a routine practice for all meconium-stained infants until a large randomized controlled trial found that intubating and suctioning vigorous infants born through MSAF had no benefit and increased the rate of complications [34]. This finding has been confirmed by additional, well-designed studies [35], prompting a change in practice guidelines in 2000. And recently, in the last quarter of 2015, ILCOR changed the ongoing practice of immediate endotracheal suctioning of the depressed infant (<100 beats per minute), poor muscle tone, and no spontaneous respiratory effort before positive pressure ventilation with prompt initiation of ventilation support. Intubation is considered when there is airway obstruction with no special relevance to MSAF [3].

Most of the infants with MSAF do not exhibit any sign of respiratory distress, but MAS can result in respiratory distress of varying severity immediately after birth or in the transition period. Umbilical cord staining takes 15 minutes with thick meconium and 1 hour with light meconium. Four-to-six-hour exposure leads to staining of nails, while nearly 12 hours are needed for vernix caseosa staining [36].

Large amounts of thick meconium can result in airway obstruction, which results in apneic or gasping respirations at first, and then as it is driven down to distal airways, respiratory distress secondary to increased resistance, decreased compliance, and air trapping develop [36].

Arterial blood gas is hypoxemic. In mild cases, hyperventilation may result in respiratory alkalosis, while in severe ones, just the opposite is true with respiratory acidosis progressing into mixed acidosis.

The typical chest radiograph initially appears streaky with diffuse parenchymal infiltrates (**Figure 2c**). In time, lungs become hyperinflated with patchy areas of atelectasis, due to inactivated surfactant by the bile acids within the meconium, and alveolar distension. Pneumomediastinum, pneumothorax, and PPHN are common in MAS [1].

Pulmonary hypertension commonly develops in severe cases and should be aggressively treated. Echocardiography helps confirm PPHN.

3.6. Pneumothorax

Pneumothorax is an abnormal accumulation of air or gas between the visceral and parietal pleura. It develops secondary to an underlying disease process such as pneumonia, meconium aspiration, ventilation, or congenital abnormalities of the lungs. It can also occur spontaneously in 1% of newborns around the perinatal period, although only about 10% of these are symptomatic [37]. On the other hand, traumatic pneumothorax can occur due to either positive pressure ventilation (PPV) or accidental insult during a central line placement [38]. Tension pneumothorax is the life-threatening condition, requiring immediate medical attention and intervention. When the air is trapped in the pleural cavity and lung volume is decreased and increased pleural pressure causes a mediastinal shift [38].

Patients with TTN, RDS, MAS, pneumonia, pulmonary hypoplasia, urinary tract anomalies, perinatal asphyxia, and infants who were resuscitated at birth or infants receiving CPAP, PPV cardiopulmonary resuscitation, and male infants are under risk [38].

The clinical presentation may vary from mild or severe signs of respiratory distress to a gradual decline in respiratory function. In non-tension pneumothorax, signs can be variable in severity such as mild-to-moderate tachypnea, apnea, irritability, grunting, pallor, and cyanosis. In tension pneumothorax, clinical findings are very severe with definite cyanosis, hypoxia, tachypnea, a sudden decrease in heart rate with bradycardia, a sudden increase in systolic blood pressure followed by narrowing pulse pressure and hypotension, an asymmetric chest, decreased breath sounds, and shift of the cardiac apical pulse away from the affected side [38].

Blood gas can reveal hypercarbia and hypoxia with respiratory acidosis and metabolic acidosis, which may accompany in tension pneumothorax.

Anteroposterior chest radiography may show shift of the mediastinum away from the affected side, depression of the diaphragm on the same side, and displacement of the lung on the

http://dx.doi.org/10.5772/64397

affected side away from the chest wall by a radiolucent band of air (**Figure 2d**). In cases of confusion, lateral decubitus view will detect even a small pneumothorax. The infant should be positioned so the side of the suspected pneumothorax is up [38].

4. Management of respiratory distress

4.1. Stepwise approach for newborn infants with respiratory distress in the delivery room

AHA guideline for neonatal resuscitation should be followed for newborns who need resuscitation in the delivery room [3]. In 2015 update, there were major management differences and new recommendations compared to 2010 guideline [3].

Spontaneously, breathing preterm infants with respiratory distress may be supported with CPAP initially rather than with routine intubation for administering PPV.

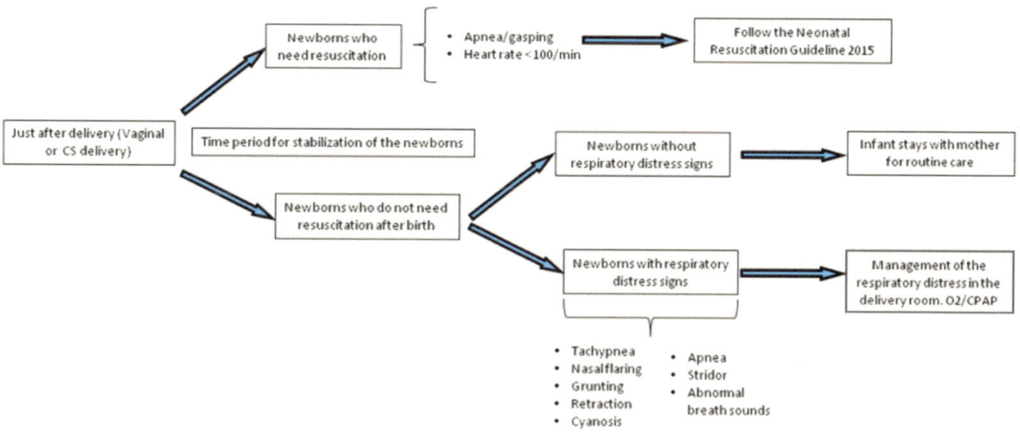

Figure 3. Practical AUCH approach for newborns in the delivery room. CS: cesarean section; AUCH: Ankara University Children's Hospital.

Practical approach for spontaneously breathing infants who do not need resuscitation but have respiratory distress signs—that is to say labored breathing (tachypnea, apnea, grunting, flaring of the nostrils, retractions) or persistent cyanosis in relevance with ILCOR 2015—in the delivery room at Ankara University Children Hospital (AUCH) is summarized in **Figures 3** and **4** . Delivered oxygen concentration to reach the targeted saturation and gestational age is a key point for practical approach to newborns with respiratory distress in our delivery room (**Figure 4**). For some newborns whose respiratory distress improves, follow-up is continued up to 20 minutes of life in the delivery room. If their respiratory signs worsen or not resolve after 20 minutes, infants should be admitted to the transitional care. On the other hand, if the infants ≥34 weeks gestation and otherwise healthy whom respiratory distress improve (the absence of clinical sign of respiratory distress, transcutaneous oxygen saturation of >90% without oxygen, respiratory rate < 60/min) within 2 hours in the transitional care unites, they can stay with the mother.

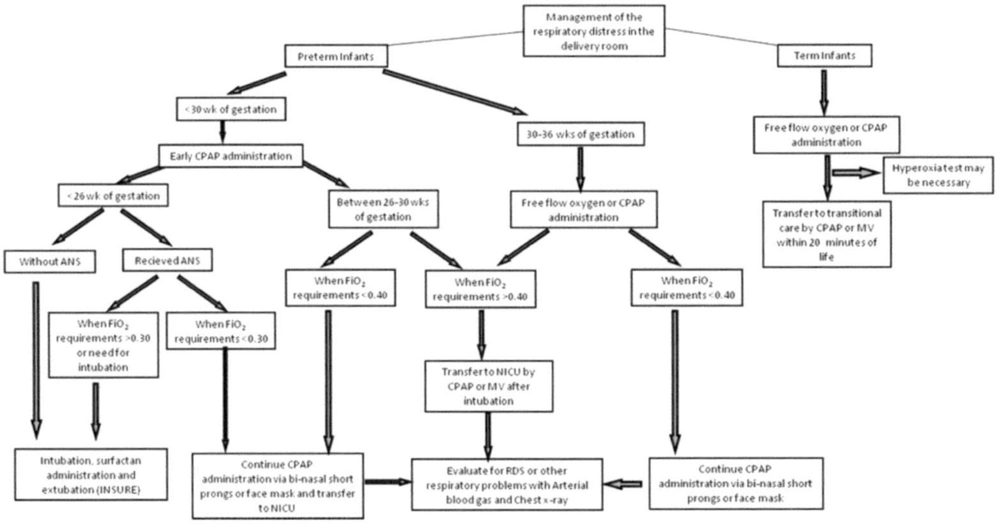

Figure 4. Practical AUCH approach for spontaneously breathing infants who have respiratory distress signs (tachypnea, apnea, grunting, flaring of the nostrils, retractions, cyanosis, etc.). AUCH: Ankara University Children's Hospital; CPAP: continuous positive airway pressure; ANS: antenatal steroid; FiO_2, fraction of inspired oxygen; MV: mechanical ventilation; NICU: neonatal intensive care unit; RDS: respiratory distress syndrome.

4.2. Treatment modalities for newborn infant's respiratory distress in the NICU

Infants with respiratory distress may need only supplemental oxygen, whereas those with respiratory distress and apnea require non-invasive or invasive mechanical ventilation [2]. Although the survival of infants with respiratory problems has dramatically improved with the treatment modalities, they may also lead to harmful side effects especially for immature infants. Avoiding lung injury and adverse effects of these treatments is the main challenge for the modern NICUs. Flow chart for newborns with respiratory distress who need assisted ventilation or who are in recovery period in our NICU is showed in **Figure 5**.

Oxygen treatment with hoods, face mask, and nasal cannulas is commonly used in the delivery room and NICUs to achieve targeted SpO_2 values or to decrease WOB. Very mild cases of respiratory distress may be successfully managed by 21–30% ambient O_2 in the incubators [2]. Optimizing oxygenation allows efficient use of respiratory muscles. Any sign of increased WOB or increasing oxygen requirement more than 40% suggests the need for early institution of positive pressure support. Babies should not be allowed to become significantly acidotic (pH<7.25) without escalating support [39].

http://dx.doi.org/10.5772/64397

Oxygen is a therapeutic gas, and insufficient or excessive oxygen can be harmful for all newborns. A non-invasive monitoring device to measure oxygen saturation by pulse oximetry should be used continuously in infants, especially in preterm ones receiving any supplemental oxygen. Although, in preterm babies receiving oxygen, the saturation target should be between 90% and 95%, the appropriate saturation ranges remain controversial [15]. Both lower (85–89%) and higher (91–95%) oxygen-saturation targets have been associated with severe morbidity and mortality in preterm infants. More recently, the trial from the BOOST-II Australia and the United Kingdom Collaborative Groups concluded that the use of an oxygen-saturation target range of 85–89% versus 91–95% resulted in significantly increased risks of death or disability at 2 years in infants born before 28 weeks' gestation. In addition, fluctuations in SpO_2 should be avoided in the postnatal period for avoiding retinopathy of prematurity (ROP) [15].

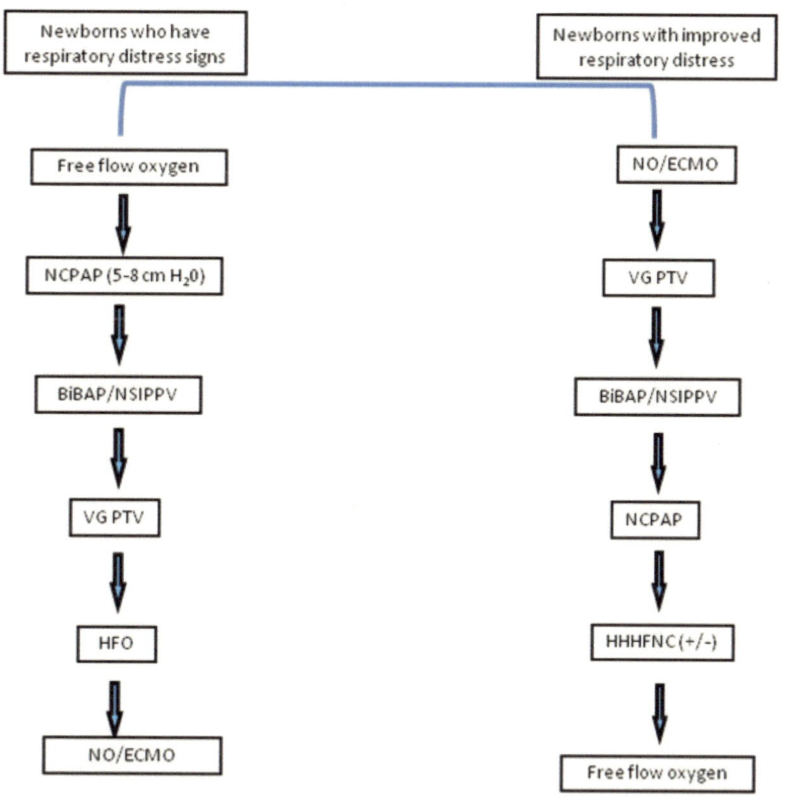

Figure 5. AUCH flow chart for newborns with respiratory distress who need assisted ventilation or who are in recovery period. NCPAP: nasal continuous positive airway pressure; BiPAP: bi-level nasal CPAP; NSIPPV: nasal synchronized intermittent positive pressure ventilation; VG PTV: volume-guarantee patient triggered ventilation; HFO: high frequency oscillatory ventilation; ECMO: extra corporeal membrane oxygenation.

Non-invasive ventilation (NIV) support can be defined as any form of respiratory support that is not delivered through an endotracheal tube [40]. Nasal CPAP (nCPAP) is a well-known useful strategy for NIV[34] [15]. Among new modes of NIV, alternating nasal positive pressures in the form of either nasal intermittent positive pressure ventilation (NIPPV) or bi-level nasal CPAP and heated humidified high-flow nasal cannula (HHHFNC) gain increasing popularity [41].

CPAP provides stabilization of the airway and allows alveolar recruitment. Flow for CPAP delivery can be continuous or variable. A warmed and humidified gas is continuously provided by ventilators and bubble CPAP devices. Infant flow CPAP system device allows expiration, provides variable flow, and reduces WOB [2].

Nasal CPAP provides end-expiratory pressure, which reduces atelectasis, maintains higher FRC, and improves lung function by reducing workload and minimizing ventilation/perfusion (V/Q) mismatch. It reduces obstructive and central apnea and improves synchronization of respiratory movements. If there is evolving signs of respiratory distress, nCPAP is best used early rather than waiting for babies to deteriorate and has been associated with a significant reduction in the need for intubation [39].

Recent randomized clinical trials demonstrated that, in comparison with prophylactic or early use of surfactant, the use of CPAP decreases the need for invasive mechanical ventilation (MV) and the combined outcome of death or BPD [42]. Although all randomized trials to date have shown a high rate of CPAP failure in the most immature infants (24–25 weeks' gestational age), these infants also may benefit most from this strategy [43].

CPAP should be started from birth in babies who is lower than 30 weeks' gestation if they do not need MV. The interface should be short binasal prongs or mask for delivering CPAP, and a starting pressure of 5–6 cm H_2O should be applied. According to European Consensus Guideline, CPAP with early rescue surfactant should be considered the optimal management for babies with RDS [15].

The use of very early (prophylactic) CPAP in spontaneously breathing preterm infants is already studied by multicenter large trials and recommended as described above. But, there is only one trial about the role of prophylactic CPAP administration to the late preterm and term infants who have a higher risk for TTN. It is found that prophylactic CPAP administration decreases the rate of NICU admission without any side effect in late preterm and early term infants delivered by elective C/S [44].

Nasal masks lead to less nasal trauma than short binasal prongs. CPAP of 5–7 cm H_2O is recommended. Babies with RDS need considerably higher PEEP than a baby with TTN or sepsis due to the noncompliant lungs. Excessive PEEP can lead to pneumothorax and may reduce cardiac output [2]. The increase in PEEP or O_2 requirements (especially greater than 40%) may suggest the further escalation of therapy.

Clinical report from the Committee on fetus and newborn for non-invasive respiratory support concluded that (a) synchronized NIPPV reduces the frequency of postextubation failure than NCPAP. (b) There is no difference between nonsynchronized NIPPV and BiPAP for postextubation failure. (c) Data do not support the advantage of NIPPV/BiPAP over nCPAP for the management of babies with RDS. (d) There is no published evidence of benefit of NIPPV or

BiPAP for apnea of prematurity. (e) Committee suggest that further research is needed before recommending NIPPV or BiPAP instead of nCPAP in RDS or apnea [41].

Heated humidified high flow nasal cannula devices used in preterm neonates should precondition inspiratory gases close to normal tracheal gas conditions (37°C and 100% relative humidity) without causing the excessive airway drying, mucosal damage, bleeding, and increased risk of infection that can complicate conventional high flow nasal oxygen. Committee on fetus and newborn also suggested that HHHFNC devices that precondition the inspiratory gas mixture and deliver 2–8 L/minute flow may be an effective alternative to nCPAP for postextubation failure. Unlike CPAP, HHHFNC can cause unpredictably high nasopharyngeal pressures and may lead to traumatic injury in the airways of the infants. An appropriate size of the prongs, detection of an adequate air leak between the prongs and the nares, and using air flow rates as low as possible will reduce the risk of harmful effects of HHHFNC [39, 41]. Despite its emerging popularity, the evidence that HHHFNC is as effective as nCPAP is largely anecdotal or retrospective [39].

In our NICU, primary modes of respiratory support are nCPAP, BiPAP, or NIPPV for infants who have spontaneous breaths. In our daily practice, infants with signs of respiratory distress as tachypnea, grunting, retractions, or need of FiO_2 greater than 21% at 20 minutes were started nCPAP (5–7 cm H_2O) in the delivery room and transferred to NICU on nCPAP. They were kept on nCPAP unless they required nCPAP >7 cm H_2O or FiO_2 ≥0.4 and if so, their positive pressure respiratory support was switched to BiPAP with the same device. BiPAP was started as 5 and 8 cm H_2O for the lower and higher CPAP levels, respectively. BiPAP pressures were increased to maximum of 7 and 10 cm H_2O for the lower and higher CPAP levels, respectively, and the pressure exchange rate was increased to maximum of 40 per minute for clinical stability and a blood gas analysis within normal ranges. Treatment is usually escalated to NIPPV if the need for FiO_2 of more than 0.4, or respiratory acidosis (pH ≤7.25), or insufficient respiratory effort, or excessive work of breathing before intubation. After de-escalation of NIV support, it was stopped when patients showed no signs of respiratory distress with nCPAP of 4 cm H_2O and BiPAP of 6–4 cm H_2O and FiO_2 <0.30.

The pressure gradient between the airway opening and lungs generated through mechanical ventilation produces a flow of gas into the lung. Conventional ventilators for newborns are either pressure or volume controlled ones [6].

Pressure-controlled ventilators deliver a preset peak inspiratory pressure (PIP), thus delivering a variable tidal volume depending largely on lung compliance. A constant flow of gas passes through the ventilator. Pressure is limited to the desired magnitude. This ventilation is usually used with the technique of synchronized intermittent mandatory ventilation (SIMV), which allows spontaneous breathing between ventilator breaths [6] and patient triggered ventilation (PTV).

Volume-controlled ventilators deliver a preset tidal volume with a variable PIP, depending largely on lung compliance. When this gas has been delivered by the piston, inspiration is terminated. Infants' tidal volume is set between 4 and 8 ml/kg. PIP may change in response to patient's effort, and historically, this mode of ventilation was not safe enough for neonates.

However, in the volume-guarantee (VG) modes, the clinician sets both a maximum PIP and a desired target volume for mechanical breaths. As recent evidence suggests that lung injury is most likely related to volutrauma, volume guarantee modes are being accessed in the newborn respiratory management. In addition, volume ventilation results in reductions or trend for reductions in duration of ventilation, pneumothorax, intracranial hemorrhage, and BPD [6]. In summary, it is known that lung injury is most directly related to excessive tidal volumes and, conversely, that an inadequate tidal volume increases work of breathing and promotes atelectasis and V/Q mismatch [39]. Volume targeted ventilation provides an open lung strategy and reduces the frequency of excessive tidal volumes, decreasing inadvertent hyperventilation. There has not, however, been conclusive evidence of improved long-term outcomes [39].

High-frequency ventilation (HFV) refers to various ventilator strategies and devices designed to provide ventilation at rapid rates and very low tidal volumes. Rates during HFV are expressed in hertz (Hz). There are two types of high frequency ventilators (high frequency jet ventilator – HFJV and high frequency oscillatory ventilator – HFOV), which are frequently used in neonatal medicine. Oscillatory ventilation is unique because exhalation is actively generated, as opposed to other forms of high frequency ventilation, in which it is passive [6].

Cochrane 2015 analysis revealed that the evidence to use elective HFOV instead of conventional ventilation for reduction in the risk of BPD is small, and the evidence is weakened by inconsistency of this effect across trials. In addition, the benefit could be counteracted by an increased risk of acute air leak [45]. More recently, Iscan et al. suggested that HFOV with a VG option resulted in constant tidal volume delivery and less fluctuant CO_2 levels compared to HFOV alone in premature infants with RDS [46].

One approach to minimize ventilator-induced lung injury is to tolerate higher levels of pCO_2 (permissive hypercapnia), allowing the use of lower tidal volumes. Unfortunately, prospective trials have not demonstrated a reduction in BPD. On the other hand, low pCO_2 is known to decrease cerebral blood flow. There is a proven association between hypocapnia, neonatal brain injury, and subsequent cerebral palsy. Hypocapnia should therefore be avoided in ventilated infants wherever possible [39].

In our NICU, preferred modes of invasive ventilatory support are volume guarantee-PTV for preterm and term infants to maintain more stable pCO_2 and to avoid over distension and subsequent volutrauma. HFOV is preferred as a rescue strategy, but it is the primary mode for CDH.

There are several different surfactant preparations that have been used in neonates with RDS, including synthetic (protein-free) and natural (derived from animal lungs) products. Natural surfactants are superior to synthetic preparations at reducing pulmonary air leaks and mortality [15]. Natural surfactants contain the hydrophobic surfactant protein, SpB and SpC, although at different concentrations. However, some synthetic surfactant preparations contain only phospholipids [2]. According to Cochrane review, in a trial comparing protein containing synthetic surfactants compared to protein-free synthetic surfactant for the prevention of RDS, no statistically different clinical differences in death and BPD were noted [47].

Some trials, which aim to compare the effect of poractant alfa and the beractant for rescue therapy, demonstrated that more rapid improvement in oxygenation was achieved with poractant alfa [15]. According to European Consensus Guideline, 200 mg/kg dose of poractant alfa has an advantage for overall survival than 100 mg/kg of beractant or 100 mg/kg of poractant alfa to treat RDS [15].

Infants receiving INSURE (intubate, surfactant, extubate) have less need for mechanical ventilation, fewer pneumothorax, and less BPD, but evidence of long-term benefit is limited.

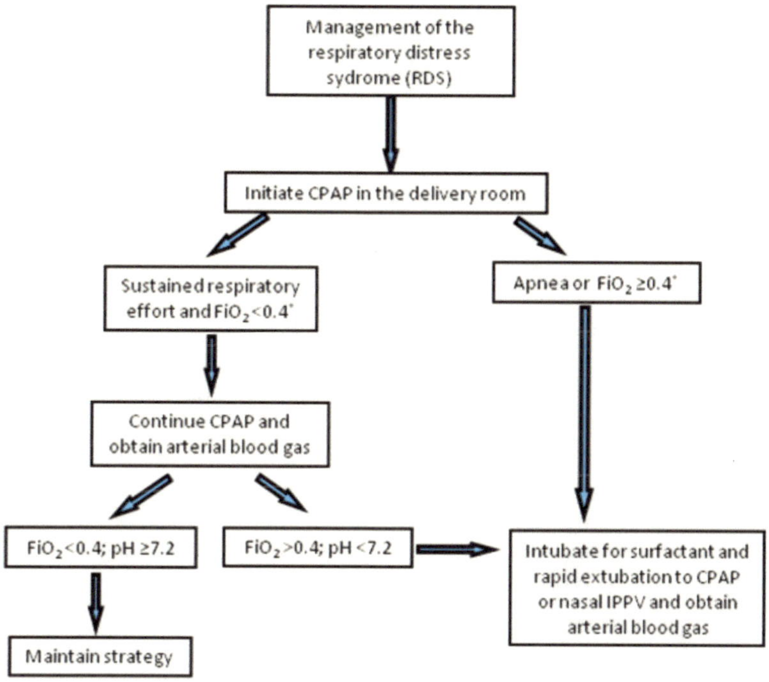

Figure 6. *FiO_2 cut off <0.3 for infants born <26 weeks of gestation. Adapted and modified from Kalus & Fanaroff's Care of the High Risk Neonate.

According to European Consensus Guideline [15]:

1. Infants diagnosed with RDS should be given a natural surfactant preparation.
2. Extremely preterm infants in whom the mother has not had antenatal steroids and infants who require intubation for stabilization surfactant should be administered in the delivery room. Except these situations, early rescue surfactant should be standard.
3. Infants with RDS should be given rescue surfactant as early as possible. A suggested protocol from European Consensus Guideline would be to treat infants <26 weeks' gestation when FiO_2 needs >0.30 and infants >26 weeks' gestation when FiO_2 needs >0.40.
4. When the initial dose of poractant alfa is 200 mg/kg, it would be better for treatment of RDS comparing to 100 mg/kg of poractant alfa or beractant.

5. Consideration of the INSURE technique is important. Because more mature babies can often be extubated to NIV just after surfactant administration, and a clinical judgment needs to be made as to whether an individual infant will tolerate this.

6. If there is evidence of ongoing RDS, a second or sometimes a third dose of surfactant can be administered.

Management of RDS in AUCH has been summarized in **Figure 6**.

There are some limited data about surfactant therapy for disease other than RDS. Preliminary reports of surfactant therapy have been noted in cases of pneumonia, pulmonary hemorrhage, MAS, and PPHN. However, an established protocol for these situations is not present [2].

Extra corporeal membrane oxygenation (ECMO) provides oxygen delivery, carbon dioxide removal, and cardiac support in patients who have cardiac and/or respiratory failure. ECMO is used for critically ill term and late preterm infants (≥32–34 weeks or ≥1.6–1.8 kg) as a rescue bridge therapy for severe but reversible respiratory and/or cardiac insufficiency in case of failure of other conventional therapies [48].

Nitric oxide (NO) is a colorless gas with a half-life of seconds stimulates soluble guanylate cyclase (sGC) to increase intracellular cGMP, which indirectly decreases the free cytosolic calcium, resulting in smooth muscle relaxation. Excess iNO diffuses into the blood stream, where it is rapidly inactivated by binding to hemoglobin and subsequent metabolism to nitrates and nitrites. This rapid inactivation thereby limits its action to the pulmonary vasculature [49].

Inhaled NO is licensed for only term and near-term neonates with hypoxic respiratory failure associated with clinical or echocardiographic evidence of pulmonary hypertension by the Food and Drug Administration in the USA [50]. Inhaled NO does not improve long-term surfactant function or markers of pulmonary inflammation and oxidative stress [51]. Although the use of iNO has increased over the years and this increase is mostly due to off-label use in premature infants, the treatment of preterm infants is more controversial [50].

Methylxanthines have been used as respiratory stimulants to decrease apnea of prematurity and to facilitate successful extubation [15, 39]. Methylxanthines increase minute ventilation, improve CO_2 sensitivity, decrease hypoxic depression, enhance diaphragmatic activity, and decrease periodic breathing [2].

The Caffeine for Apnea of Prematurity (CAP) study evaluated the issue of long-term effects of caffeine therapy in infants who were under 1250 g birth weight. Study infants randomly had caffeine or placebo in the first 10 days of life and continuing until the clinician decision. Babies in caffeine group weaned off ventilation a week earlier and had significant reduction in BPD than placebo group [15]. According to CAP study, the combined outcome of death or neurodisability decreased in caffeine-treated babies at 18 months and also reduced rates of cerebral palsy and cognitive delay [52]. The differences were no longer significant after 5 years but reassuring that there were no long-term adverse effects on development. Infants who were on MV and had started caffeine earliest appeared to provide the most benefit [52].

Author details

Begüm Atasay[1*], İlke Mungan Akın[2] and Serdar Alan[3]

*Address all correspondence to: begumatasay@hotmail.com

1 Division of Neonatology, Department of Pediatrics, Ankara University, Ankara, Turkey

2 Göztepe Hospital, İstanbul Medeniyet University, İstanbul, Turkey

3 Yüksek İhtisas University, Koru Sincan Hospital, Ankara, Turkey

References

[1] Reuter S, Moser C, Baack M. Respiratory distress in the newborn. Pediatr Rev. 2014;35(10):417–428. doi: 10.1542/pir.35-10-417.

[2] Respiratory management. In: Gomella TL, Cunningham MD, Eyal FG (eds.). Neonatology: Management, Procedures, On-Call Problems, Diseases, and Drugs. 7th ed. USA: Lange McGraw Hill Education LLC; 2013. pp. 71–89.

[3] Wyckoff MH, Aziz K, Escobedo MB, Kapadia VS, Kattwinkel J, Perlman JM, Simon WM, Weiner GM, Zaichkin JG. Part 13: neonatal resuscitation: 2015 American Heart Association Guidelines Update for cardiopulmonary resuscitation and emergency cardiovascular care. Circulation. 2015;132(18):543–560. doi: 10.1161/CIR.0000000000000267.

[4] Vanden Hoek TL, Morrison LJ, Shuster M, Donnino M, Sinz E, Lavonas EJ, Jeejeebhoy FM, Gabrielli A. Special Report-Neonatal Resuscitation: 2010 American Heart Association Guidelines for cardiopulmonary resuscitation and emergency cardiovascular care. Circulation. 2010;122:909–919. doi: 10.1161/CIRCULATIONAHA.110.971069.

[5] Sandberg KL, Brynjarsson H, Hjalmarson O. Transcutaneous blood gas monitoring during neonatal intensive care. Acta Paediatr. 2011;100(5):676–679. doi: 10.1111/j.1651-2227.2011.02164.x.

[6] Martin JM, Crowley MA. Respiratory problems. In: Fanaroff AA, Fanaroff JM (eds.). Klaus & Fanaroff's Care of the High Risk Neonate. 6th ed. Philadelphia: Elsevier Saunders; 2013. pp. 244–269.

[7] Jain L, Dudell GG. Respiratory transition in infants delivered by cesarean section. Semin Perinatol. 2006;30(5):296–304.

[8] Hooper SB, Kitchen MJ, Wallace MJ, et al. Imaging lung aeration and lung liquid clearance at birth. FASEB J. 2007;21(12):3329–3337.

[9] te Pas AB, Davis PG, Hooper SB, Morley CJ. From liquid to air: breathing after birth. J Pediatr. 2008;152(5):607–611. doi: 10.1016/j.jpeds.2007.10.041.

[10] Atasay B, Ergun H, Okulu E, Mungan Akın I, Arsan S. The association between cord hormones and transient tachypnea of newborn in late preterm and term neonates who were delivered by cesarean section. J Matern Fetal Neonatal Med. 2013;26(9):877–880. doi: 10.3109/14767058.2013.765846.

[11] Milner A, Saunders R, Hopkins I. Effects of delivery by cesarean section on lung mechanics and lung volume in the human neonate. Arch Dis Childhood. 1978;53:545–548.

[12] Dani C, Reali MF, Bertini G, Wiechmann L, Spagnolo A, Tangucci M, et al. Risk factors for the development of respiratory distress syndrome and transient tachypnea in newborn infants. Italian Group of Neonatal Pneumology. Eur Respir J. 1999;14:155–159.

[13] Clark JM, Hulme E, Devendrakumar V, Turner MA, Baker PN, Sibley CP, et al. Effect of maternal asthma on birth weight and neonatal outcome in a British inner-city population. Paediatr Perinatal Epidemiol. 2007;21:154–162.

[14] Gouyon J, Ribakovsky C, Ferdynus C, Quantin C, Sagot P, Gouyon B. Severe respiratory disorders in term neonates. Paediatr Perinatal Epidemiol. 2007;22:22–30. doi: 10.1111/j.1365-3016.2007.00875.x.

[15] Sweet DG, Carnielli V, Greisen G, Hallman M, Ozek E, Plavka R, Saugstad OD, Simeoni U, Speer CP, Vento M, Halliday HL; European Association of Perinatal Medicine. European Consensus Guidelines on the management of neonatal respiratory distress syndrome in preterm ınfants – update 2013. Neonatology. 2013;103(4):353–368. doi: 10.1159/000349928.

[16] Transient tachypnea of the newborn. In: Gomella TL, Cunningham MD, Eyal FG (eds.). Neonatology: Management, Procedures, On-Call Problems, Diseases, and Drugs. 7th ed. USA: Lange McGraw Hill Education LLC; 2013. pp. 947–954.

[17] Rubaltelli FF, Dani C, Reali MF, Bertini G, Wiechmann L, Tangucci M, Spagnolo A. Acute neonatal respiratory distress in Italy: a one year prospective study, Italian Group of Neonatal Pneumology. Acta Paediatr. 1998;87(12):1261–1268.

[18] Weisman LE, Hansen TN. Contemporary Diagnosis and Management of Neonatal Respiratory Diseases. 3rd ed. Newton, PA: Handbooks in Health Care Co.; 2003, Chapter 4.

[19] Edwards MO, Kotecha SJ, Kotecha S. Respiratory distress of the term newborn infant. Paediatr Respir Rev. 2013;14(1):29–36. doi: 10.1016/j.prrv.2012.02.002.

[20] Verani JR, McGee L, Schrag SJ. Division of Bacterial Diseases, National Center for Immunization and Respiratory Diseases, Centers for Disease Control and Prevention.

Prevention of perinatal group B streptococcal disease: revised guidelines from CDC, 2010. MMWR Recomm Rep. 2010;59(RR-10):1–36.

[21] Randis TM, Polin RA. Early-onset group B streptococcal sepsis: new recommendations from the Centres for Disease Control and Prevention. Arch Dis Child Fetal Neonatal Ed. 2012;97(4):F291–F294. doi: 10.1136/archdischild-2011-300627.

[22] Cleveland RH. A radiologic update on medical diseases of the newborn chest. Pediatr Radiol. 1995;25:631–7.

[23] Respiratory distress syndrome. In: Gomella TL, Cunningham MD, Eyal FG (eds.) Neonatology: Management, Procedures, On-Call Problems, Diseases, and Drugs. 7th ed. USA: Lange McGraw Hill Education LLC; 2013. pp. 868–872.

[24] Sweet DG, Carnielli V, Greisen G, Hallman M, Ozek E, Plavka R, et al. European consensus guidelines on the management of neonatal respiratory distress syndrome in preterm infants – 2010 update. Neonatology. 2010;97:402–417. doi: 10.1159/000297773.

[25] Roberts D, Dalziel S. Antenatal corticosteroids for accelerating fetal lung maturation for women at risk of preterm birth. Cochrane Database Syst Rev. 2006;19(3):CD004454.

[26] Crowther CA, McKinlay CJ, Middleton P, Harding JE. Repeat doses of prenatal corticosteroids for women at risk of preterm birth for improving neonatal health outcomes. Cochrane Database Syst Rev. 2011;15(6):CD003935. doi: 10.1002/14651858.CD003935.pub3.

[27] Kenyon S, Boulvain M, Neilson JP. Antibiotics for preterm rupture of membranes. Cochrane Database Syst Rev. 2010;4(8):CD001058. doi: 10.1002/14651858.CD001058.pub2.

[28] Haas DM, Caldwell DM, Kirkpatrick P, McIntosh JJ, Welton NJ. Tocolytic therapy for preterm delivery: systematic review and network meta-analysis. BMJ. 2012;345:e6226. doi: 10.1136/bmj.e6226.

[29] Persistent pulmonary hypertension of the newborn. In: Gomella TL, Cunningham MD, Eyal FG (eds.). Neonatology: Management, Procedures, On-Call Problems, Diseases, and Drugs. 7th ed. USA: Lange McGraw Hill Education LLC; 2013. pp. 843–851.

[30] Kotecha S, Barbato A, Bush A, Claus F, Davenport M, Delacourt C, et al. European respiratory society task force on congenital diaphragmatic hernia. Eur Respir J. 2012;39(4):820–829. doi: 10.1183/09031936.00066511.

[31] Yeh TF. Meconium aspiration syndrome: pathogenesis and current management. Neoreviews. 2010;11:e503–e551. doi: 10.1542/neo.11-9-e503.

[32] Gülmezoglu AM, Crowther CA, Middleton P, Heatley E. Induction of labour for improving birth outcomes for women at or beyond term. Cochrane Database Syst Rev. 2012;6:CD004945. doi: 10.1002/14651858.CD004945.pub3.

[33] Fraser WD, Hofmeyr J, Lede R, et al. Amnioinfusion for the prevention of the meconium aspiration syndrome. N Engl J Med. 2005;353(9):909–917.

[34] Linder N, Aranda JV, Tsur M, et al. Need for endotracheal intubation and suction in meconium-stained neonates. J Pediatr. 1988;112(4):613–615.

[35] Wiswell TE, Gannon CM, Jacob J, et al. Delivery room management of the apparently vigorous meconium-stained neonate: results of the multicenter, international collaborative trial. Pediatrics. 2000;105(1, pt 1):1–7.

[36] Meconium aspiration. In: Gomella TL, Cunningham MD, Eyal FG (eds.) Neonatology: Management, Procedures, On-Call Problems, Diseases, and Drugs. 7th ed. USA: Lange McGraw Hill Education LLC; 2013. pp. 777–782.

[37] Greenough A, Morley C, Roberton N. Acute respiratory diseases in the newborn. In: Roberton N (ed.). Textbook of Neonatology. 2nd ed. London: Churchill Livingstone; 1992. pp. 385–504.

[38] Pneumothorax. In: Gomella TL, Cunningham MD, Eyal FG (eds.). Neonatology: Management, Procedures, On-Call Problems, Diseases, and Drugs. 7th ed. USA: Lange McGraw Hill Education LLC; 2013. pp. 502–508.

[39] BOOST-II Australia and United Kingdom Collaborative Groups. Outcomes of two trials of oxygen-saturation targets in preterm infants. N Engl J Med. 2016;374(8):749–760. doi: 10.1056/NEJMoa1514212. [Epub ahead of print]

[40] Cummings JJ, Polin RA; Committee on Fetus and Newborn. Noninvasive respiratory support. Pediatrics. 2016;137(1):1–11. doi: 10.1542/peds.2015-3758.

[41] Fischer HS, Bührer C. Avoiding endotracheal ventilation to prevent bronchopulmonary dysplasia: a meta-analysis. Pediatrics. 2013;132(5):e1351–e1360. doi: 10.1542/peds.2013-1880.

[42] Schmölzer GM, Kumar M, Pichler G, Aziz K, O'Reilly M, Cheung PY. Non-invasive versus invasive respiratory support in preterm infants at birth: systematic review and meta-analysis. BMJ. 2013;347(347):f5980. doi: 10.1136/bmj.f5980.

[43] Carlo WA, Finer NN, Walsh MC, et al. Target ranges of oxygen saturation in extremely preterm infants. N Engl J Med. 2010;362(21):1959–1969. doi: 10.1056/NEJMoa0911781.

[44] Keszler M. State of the art in conventional mechanical ventilation. J Perinatol. 2009;29:262–275. doi: 10.1038/jp.2009.11.

[45] Cools F, Offringa M, Askie LM. Elective high frequency oscillatory ventilation versus conventional ventilation for acute pulmonary dysfunction in preterm infants. Cochrane Database Syst Rev. 2015;19(3):CD000104. doi: 10.1002/14651858.CD000104.pub4.

[46] Iscan B, Duman N, Tuzun F, Kumral A, Ozkan H. Impact of volume guarantee on high-frequency oscillatory ventilation in preterm infants: a randomized crossover clinical trial. Neonatology. 2015;108(4):277–282. doi: 10.1159/000437204.

[47] Pfister RH, Soll R, Wiswell TE. Protein-containing synthetic surfactant versus protein-free synthetic surfactant for the prevention and treatment of respiratory distress syndrome. Cochrane Database Syst Rev. 2009;7(4):CD006180. doi: 10.1002/14651858.CD006180.pub2.

[48] Carlo WA, Ambalavanan N. Assisted ventilation. In: Fanaroff AA, Fanaroff JM (eds.). Klaus & Fanaroff's Care of the High Risk Neonate. 6th ed. Philadelphia: Elsevier Saunders; 2013. pp. 270–288.

[49] Clark RH, Ursprung RL, Walker MW, Ellsbury DL, Spitzer AR. The changing pattern of inhaled nitric oxide use in the neonatal intensive care unit. J Perinatol. 2010;30(12): 800–804. doi: 10.1038/jp.2010.37.

[50] Ballard PL, Merrill JD, Truog WE, Godinez RI, Godinez MH, McDevitt TM, et al. Surfactant function and composition in premature infants treated with inhaled nitric oxide. Pediatrics. 2007;120:346–353.

[51] Ballard PL, Truog WE, Merrill JD, Gow A, Posencheg M, Golombek SG, et al. Plasma biomarkers of oxidative stress: relationship to lung disease and inhaled nitric oxide therapy in premature infants. Pediatrics. 2008;121:555–561. doi: 10.1542/peds. 2007-2479.

[52] Schmidt B, Anderson PJ, Doyle LW, Dewey D, Grunau RE, Asztalos EV, Davis PG, Tin W, Moddemann D, Solimano A, Ohlsson A, Barrington KJ, Roberts RS, Caffeine for Apnea of Prematurity (CAP) Trial Investigators. Survival without disability to age 5 years after neonatal caffeine therapy for apnea of prematurity. JAMA. 2012;307:275–282. doi: 10.1001/jama.2011.2024.

Chapter 8

Perinatal Lung Development: The Lung at Birth

Jyh-Chang Jean, Lou Ann Scism Brown and
Martin Joyce-Brady

Additional information is available at the end of the chapter

http://dx.doi.org/10.5772/63819

Abstract

The successful transition from liquid to air breathing at birth is essential in mammalian lung development and the primary biological role of the hypothalamic-pituitary-adrenal axis. At this moment, the lung experiences a major environmental change in oxygen tension as the fluid that filled this organ in utero (pO2 ~26) is rapidly replaced with ambient air during the first few breaths (pO2 ~150). This change induces oxidant stress in the lung which is balanced by antioxidant genes that are induced in the late gestational fetal lung to protect against injury. These antioxidant genes impact distinct antioxidant molecules, including glutathione, which can regulate the level of redox stress in lung cells. Cells, such as the alveolar macrophage, are central for host defense and surfactant homeostasis at the newly established air-liquid surface. Yet they are prone to dysfunction with excessive oxidant stress and the newborn lung is susceptible to infection. And yet the rise in alveolar oxygen tension can also serve as a physiologic redox signal that initiates expression of genes that regulate postnatal lung development. Taken together, birth can be viewed as a natural experiment with hyperoxia where the birth process itself serves as an integrator for that level of redox stress that limits lung injury while activating genes required for postnatal lung development.

Keywords: lung, perinatal, birth shock, glutathione, Kruppel-like factor 4

1. Introduction

The symbols for man (♂), woman (♀), birth (✲), death (†), and infinity (∞) were penned on a blackboard at the opening of the 1960s medical drama "Ben Casey." These symbols represented a fundamental organization of life in the universe of medicine. Birth was a culmination of a progressive series of molecular and cellular events that began with fertilization, progressed through gastrulation, and then embryogenesis to form the fetus and finally the newborn child. Along the way, an ever enlarging population of cells proliferated, migrated, differentiated, and died and a host of organs with unique functions were constructed on organ-specific extracellular matrices connected to each other by vessels and to the external environment by tubes. Herein, we focus on a select aspect of lung development in the perinatal period. At that time, the fetus experienced a unique transition from a highly protected fluid-filled uterine environment to a highly susceptible gas-filled environment that marked its independent existence as a newborn. The role of the lung as a secretory organ came to an end and its new role as a gas exchanger began. In so doing, the cells of the lung, more so than any other organ, were immediately exposed to an elevated concentration of oxygen.

Decades of lung developmental research have unraveled many features about lung function in the perinatal period. Some highlights include a primary role for hormones in regulating lung cell maturation along with the ontogeny of a surfactant lipoglycoprotein complex to ensure the success of this transition, particularly the hypothalamic-pituitary-adrenal axis [1]. Although some aspects of perinatal lung alveolar, cell surface differentiation is steroid-independent [2]. Identification of regulators that control the progression of lung progenitor cells into distinct lineages to form distal lung alveolar cells [3]. The molecular events occurring during lung development are regulated by transcription factors, and the families involved are extensive [3, 4]. In this review, we will focus on a particular transcription factor family known as the Kruppel-like factors (KLF). Krüppel is a zinc-finger transcription factor described in *Drosophila melanogaster* as essential for pattern formation and embryogenesis [5]. A related family of mammalian Krüppel-like factors, Klfs, share sequence homology with the DNA-binding domain of Krüppel and serve essential roles in mammalian embryogenesis [6]. Lung Kruppel-like factor, Klf2, has been known to be important in lung development [7]. Another member, Klf5, was shown more recently to play a role in perinatal lung development [8]. Interestingly, Klf5 is known to interact with Klf4, gut enriched Kruppel-like factor, which we will highlight in this review [9].

2. The Kruppel-like family of transcription factors and the lung

Lung development is characterized by a dramatic structural and functional re-organization from an organ of secretion *in utero* to one of the gas exchanges at birth. This morphologic transition is only partially complete in the newborn murine and human lung. The process of forming new alveoli in the lung occurs largely in the postnatal period. It involves regulation of cell proliferation, differentiation, migration, and apoptosis and affects epithelial, endothelial, and interstitial cell populations within the lung parenchyma and airways. It also involves complex interactions between cells and extracellular matrix proteins [10]. Previous literature described many of the cellular components of these critical postnatal events, and contemporary research has concentrated on the molecular regulators that drive the formation of the gas exchange surface and the mechanical properties of the postnatal lung.

http://dx.doi.org/10.5772/63819

It was known that there was a progressive decline in cell proliferation in mesenchymal cells, including fibroblasts [11] and epithelial cells [12, 13], near the end of gestation, at birth, and during the early postnatal period. The effect was transient as the number of proliferating cells rose dramatically in the late postnatal period with the onset of alveolarization and continued over the next 2–3 weeks [14]. During this time, the interstitium, which was thick and packed with cells at birth, became progressively more thin and sparse with maturation of the alveolar wall [15]. The relative number of interstitial cells actually declined.

Fibroblast differentiation after birth was believed to serve major function in forming alveoli in the late postnatal lung. A population of myofibroblasts, located at the tips of developing septa, expressed α-smooth muscle actin (α-SMA) and produced matrix proteins such as elastin. The location of these cells denoted sites of newly forming alveoli and alveolarization extended from postnatal day 5 through day 20 in the mouse lung. This ability to form new alveoli appeared to be dependent upon the response of the myofibroblast to certain stimuli such as FGF-3, FGF-4 [16], and PDGF-A [17] receptors, as well as deposited matrix protein [18, 19] and transforming growth factor (TGF)-β activity, including a component of the TGF-β signaling pathway, Smad3 [20, 21]. Myofibroblasts are believed to re-emerge *de novo* in adult lung following tissue injury [22] and are postulated to play a role in repair. Differentiated fibroblasts also produce matrix proteins, including elastin and collagen. The lung actually has very little connective tissue at birth. As a result, lung elastic recoil is limited and the lung is prone to rupture by applied pressure. Production of matrix proteins such as elastin and collagen by interstitial fibroblasts during alveolarization contributes to elasticity and structural integrity to the lung [23]. Interestingly, regulation of cell proliferation and cell differentiation is a role that is reiterated in much of the Kruppel family literature.

Overall, the Kruppel-like family currently consists of over 16 members, and the originally descriptive nomenclature is now being revised into a numerical grouping system based on sequence homology, functional domains and transcriptional activity [24]. For instance, Klf4 is also known as EZF (epithelial zinc finger) and gut-enriched Klf (GKLF). It activates and represses gene transcription and has autoregulatory activity [25]. Klf2 is also known as lung Klf. It is mainly an activator of transcription and plays a role in blood vessel and lung development. **Table 1** summarizes selected aspects of a select Klfs and more detailed summaries are available in recent reviews [24, 26–28].

The Klfs are a subset of a larger family that includes Sp1 and Sp1-like proteins with Sp1 being the founding member of the family. Sp1 and Sp-1 like proteins are grouped together by phylogenetic tree analysis of protein sequences (group I) and the Klfs divide into groups II and III [24]. In general, Sp1 and Sp1-like members preferentially recognize the GT box in promoters (5′-GGTGTGGGG-3′), whereas the Klf members preferentially recognize the CA box (5′-CACCC-3′). However, competition among members for these sites and post-translational modifications that affect DNA-binding site affinity is an active area of investigation. It is believed that this diversity of protein members allows for a precise regulation of gene expression under a variety of physiological conditions. The ability of the Klf family to regulate cell proliferation, survival, and differentiation of different cell lineages suggests a potentially broad role in normal development, response to injury, and carcinogenesis.

Klf #	**Alternate name**	**Transcriptional activity**	**Cell functions**	**Phylogenetic grouping**	**Expression sites**	**Expressed in lung**
Klf2	Lung KLF	Activator	Blood vessel, lung development, T cell survival	II	Blood vessels, hematopoietic cells	+ [29, 30]
Klf4	Gut KLF	Activator/ repressor	Anti-proliferation Survival	II	Gut, epithelium, fibroblasts	+ [31, 32]
Klf5	BTEB2	Activator	Cell growth	II		+ [7, 33]
Klf6	COPEB	Activator	Putative tumor suppressor	II		+ [34]
Klf9	BTEB1	Activator/ repressor	Neurite outgrowth Carcinogen metabolism	III	Ubiquitous	+ [35]
Klf13	BTEB3	Activator/ repressor	Anti-proliferation Carcinogen metabolism	III		+ [36]

Table 1. Select characteristics for some members of the Krüppel-like family.

Klf4 was initially characterized in two independent laboratories. One identified it as a novel zinc-finger protein expressed in differentiated epithelial cells, hence named epithelial zinc finger (EZF) [31], and transiently in certain mesenchymal cells. The other identified it as a gut-enriched Krüppel-like factor expressed during growth arrest, hence GKLF [32]. In cultured fibroblasts, expression was abundant in growth-arrested cells and barely detectable in rapidly proliferating cells as the protein inhibited DNA synthesis. The message transcript was most abundant in colon followed by testis, lung, and small intestine by Northern blot and in epithelial cells of the colon as they migrated from the base to the top of the crypt [32]. Message was not detectable in the mouse embryo by Northern blot until day 15.5, but was evident in mesenchymal cells of the first branchial arch at day 11.5 and the metanephric kidney at day 12.5 by in situ hybridization. At day 15.5, the situ signal was detected in epithelial cells of the colon and the tongue and by the newborn period in epithelial cells of the esophagus and the stomach as well [31]. Message was also evident in skin of adult mice [31]. More recently, Klf4 expression has been defined in corneal epithelial cells [37]. This new gene was hypothesized to play a role in epithelial cells in many organs during differentiation in development and in mesenchymal cells during early formation of the skeleton and kidney.

These original studies demonstrated that Kl4 was an important regulator of cell proliferation and cell differentiation. In keeping with this concept, serum deprivation, DNA damage, and contact inhibition were associated with decreased proliferation and increased Klf4 expression [32, 38], while GI neoplastic lesions [39, 40] and cancer cell lines [41] were associated with high levels of proliferation but decreased levels of Klf4 expression. In tissues, Klf4 was expressed largely in post-mitotic, terminally differentiated epithelial cells [31, 32]. Transcriptional profiling of Klf4 confirmed this dual role in cell cycle regulation and epithelial cell differen-

http://dx.doi.org/10.5772/63819

tiation [42]. Cell cycle inhibitors were upregulated by Klf4, including the cdk inhibitor p21$^{WAF1/CIP1}$, and cell cycle activators were downregulated, including cyclinD1 [38, 43]. Targeted elimination of the Klf4 gene in mice revealed its critical role in terminal differentiation of epithelial cells in the skin in the perinatal period [44]. Loss of barrier function was lethal within 24 h of birth due to the rapid loss of fluids. An independent Klf4 gene ablation experiment not only confirmed this observation but also showed an alteration in the terminal differentiation program of epithelial goblet cells in the colon [45].

In keeping with the known expression of Klf4 in mesenchymal cells, several studies demonstrated regulation of this gene in non-epithelial cell types. Human Klf4 was originally cloned from a human umbilical vein cDNA library after the initial description of mouse Klf4 [46]. More recently, Klf4 induction was observed in a genomic analysis of immediate/early responses to shear stress in human coronary artery endothelial cells [47]. Shear stress inhibits endothelial cell proliferation, and Klf4 was postulated to provide a mechanism for this effect. Studies with cardiac fibroblasts identified Klf4 induction by DNA microarray and linked its expression with several cell cycle and differentiation-associated genes that were induced with a sudden change from hypoxic to normoxic conditions *in vitro* to model "perceived hyperoxia" of ischemia-reperfusion. Klf4 was proposed to play a role in activating pathways for growth-arrest and fibroblast differentiation in these cells in response to oxygen-induced injury [48]. Klf4 has also been shown to mediate redox-sensitive inhibition of proliferation in vascular smooth muscle cells [49]. Klf4 induction in response oxidant exposure was dependent on hydroxyl radical production, intracellular calcium, p38 MAP kinase activation, and protein synthesis, although a transcriptional mechanism for its induction was not defined. The Klf4 response was rapid, detectable within 30 min, and associated with induction of p21$^{WAF/Cip1}$, p27, and p53, known Klf4 target genes and inhibitors of cell proliferation. While Klf4 expression was known previously to respond to changes in the cell environment, this study identified oxidants as an additional extracellular signaling stimulus for Kl4 induction, and linked induction was activation of the MAPK signal transduction pathway.

Prior to our investigation, little was known about a role for Klf4 in lung development. Nonetheless, lung Klf4 expression had been reported in the lung in several different studies. The original characterizations of Klf4 noted expression in the adult [32] and the newborn lung [31]. Klf4 induction was also described in newborn compared to 4-week-old mice, a time of active lung cell proliferation and differentiation [50]. Early and transient Klf4 protein induction was described in the lung within 2 h following pneumonectomy although the cellular site was not determined [51]. Klf4 mRNA expression was induced in the airway transcriptome in response to cigarette smoke [52]. Klf4 mRNA was induced in alveolar epithelial type 1-like cells in response to ozone exposure [53]. Klf4 has very recently been shown to directly regulate TGF-β induced myofibroblast differentiation in isolated adult rat lung fibroblasts by inhibiting expression of α-SMA [54]. In this model, a Klf4 protein–protein interaction with Smad3 blocks Smad3 binding to a Smad3-binding element in the α-SMA promoter. This direct linkage of Klf4 with Smad3 reveals a novel mechanism by which Klf4 regulates TGF-β-induced myofibroblast gene expression in adult lung.

With this background in mind, our finding that lung Klf4 mRNA was dramatically upregulated with birth in a normal oxygen environment and attenuation of this induction by birth in a more hypoxic environment led us to hypothesize that Klf4 was regulated in a redox-responsive fashion in lung mesenchymal cells and that its target genes regulated fibroblast proliferation and differentiation events associated with postnatal lung development [55].

3. Oxygen as a regulator of Kruppel-like factor 4 in the newborn lung

This birth shock hypothesis was studied in time-pregnant mice by comparing findings in the lung with those with those in the liver, an organ that is not exposed to the same changes in environmental oxygen as the lung right at birth. And changes in newborn organs at 2, 6, 12, and 24 h after birth were compared with those of the corresponding fetal organ at day 21 of gestation, the time just before birth. Changes in gene expression at birth were examined with microarrays, and these data revealed an acute change in the level of expression of 157 genes within 2 h of birth in room air in the lung. The number of gene changes steadily declined at 6, 12, and 24 h thereafter. Most of the lung gene changes through 6 h involved transient induction or repression of expression. Less than 30% of the changes involved genes in common to any two successive time points, suggesting the presence of sequential waves of new gene expression over time. The full implication of this pattern is yet to be fully understood. Nonetheless, four functional categories of gene expression were overrepresented in these microarray data at 2 h after birth in room air: transcriptional regulators, structural genes, apoptosis-related genes, and antioxidants. Glutathione disulfide was analyzed to determine whether there was a change in the local redox state after birth in room air. This oxidation product accumulated fourfold within 2 h of birth and steadily decreased thereafter. Glutathione was always in excess of glutathione disulfide at all times points indicating a surfeit of antioxidant buffering capacity. But the lung is exposed to a transient oxidant stress and a change in the local redox state with the rise in environmental oxygen at birth.

Contrast these lung findings with those in the liver after birth in room air. The liver exhibited no accumulation of glutathione disulfide at the 2 h time point and no sign of oxidant stress at any of the early time points thereafter. These data suggest that the liver may not be subjected to the same magnitude of change in environmental oxygen tension as the lung at birth or it may follow a very different time course. In addition, there were far fewer changes in gene expression in the liver at 2 h after birth when compared to the lung, and no functional categories of gene expression were found to be overrepresented in the liver gene microarray dataset. There were a few gene expression levels that did change in common between these two organs. These could represent a shared response to the birth process itself. But we interpreted the majority of unique changes in the lung as a lung-specific response related to the change in alveolar oxygen content at birth.

To explore this, we examined a group of time-pregnant mice exposed to 10% oxygen using a glove bag at the 21st day of gestation. Some of these hypoxic mice were killed after 12 h to harvest fetal lung and assess baseline fetal measures at the end of gestation, whereas others were monitored and newborn lung was collected again at 2, 6, and 12 h after birth. Of note

http://dx.doi.org/10.5772/63819

here, all dams, fetuses, and newborns survived in the 10% oxygen environment, and this exposure did not significantly alter baseline gene expression in the fetal lung as determined with microarrays. This survival pattern suggested that changes in blood flow, lung stretch, nutrient supply, and fluid resorption were similar to that of mice birthed in room air and that these factors were less likely to differentially impact gene expression. Birth into 10% oxygen, however, did impact the level of redox stress in the lung at birth as well as the number of gene expression changes. Accumulation of glutathione disulfide was attenuated by half compared to the normal lung. And there was a 60% decrease in the number of gene changes at 2 h, compared to that in room air with elimination of any overrepresented functional category of gene expression. It was as if birth into an environment of hypoxia lacked any change in gene expression at all and retained a pattern like that of the fetal lung. The transient rise and fall in glutathione disulfide in the newborn lung in room air, despite the induction of several antioxidants in the late fetal lung and the lung at birth which buffered some but not all such stress [56–59], supports our hypothesis that a measured degree of redox stress, a birth shock, may serve a function in the lung at birth which we surmise is signalling expression of lung genes required for the onset of postnatal lung development [55].

The most provocative piece of data in our study was finding that the gene exhibiting the greatest change in expression in the lung at birth in room air was a transcription factor. And that transcription factor was Kruppel-like factor 4. Klf4 was previously referred to as gut Kruppel-like factor (GKLF), a tissue-specific gene that inhibited cell proliferation and stimulated differentiation in the gut, particularly in the epithelial cells of the crypts where there is a tight link between growth arrest and differentiation. Klf4 regulates cell proliferation by inhibiting cell-cycle progression and inducing growth arrest [31, 32, 60]. Mesenchymal and epithelial cell proliferation is known to progressively decline in the lung during the perinatal period [29–31], and a transcription factor like Klf4 is a reasonable candidate to regulate this process. Klf4 is known to induce growth arrest in cells through the cell-cycle inhibitor $p21^{WAF/Cip1}$, and the absence of Klf4 in the Klf4 knockout mouse is associated with a corresponding decrease in the level of $p21^{WAF/Cip1}$ mRNA expression in the late fetal lung and persistent cell proliferation in fibroblasts and airway epithelial cells at birth [55].

Klf4 has previously been described in the mesenchyme during development [31]. We generated Klf4 knockout and Klf4 expressing fibroblasts to demonstrate that smooth muscle actin, fibronectin, tenascin C, and the alpha 1 chain of Type 1 collagen are Klf4 target genes and that fibroblast connective tissue gene expression is down-regulated in the perinatal lung of the Klf4 knockout mouse [55]. Impaired connective tissue gene expression has at least two distinct biological implications for postnatal lung development. First, lack of collagen synthesis decreases the tensile strength of the postnatal lung and increases the risk for rupture under pressure [61] and emphysema [62]. Second, lack of fibronectin, type 1 collagen, tenascin C, and smooth muscle actin expression can impair myofibroblast differentiation and postnatal alveogenesis [63–66]. Interestingly, Klf4 our study confirmed differential regulation of smooth muscle actin gene expression in the myofibroblast and the vascular smooth muscle cell as Klf4 deficiency in the Klf4 knockout mouse lead to a loss of expression in the myofibroblast (positive regulator) but preservation of expression in the vascular smooth cell (negative regulator). This negative regulatory function in vascular smooth muscle cells was already known [67].

Finally, cell death was also increased in the Klf4-deficient lung of the Klf4 knockout mouse at birth. An expanding literature now describes Klf4 as an inhibitor of apoptosis [6]. Apoptosis is present even in the normal lung at birth and may play a physiologic role in postnatal lung development [68, 69]. We found an excess of apoptosis in the Klf4-deficient lung of the Klf4 knockout mouse, and this could well contribute to a loss of cell population and gene expression at birth. We also noticed that apoptosis exhibited a cell-specific rather than a general nature, as it was not increased in vascular smooth muscle cells within large blood vessels [55]. Taken together, we found good correlation between the gene categories that were overrepresented in the gene changes 2 h after birth and Klf4 as a potential regulator of these gene categories.

Is Klf4 expression in lung fibroblasts regulated by hyperoxia? We showed that it is and the mechanism is transcriptional in nature and independent of protein synthesis [55]. Further details of the mechanism await more studies. But Klf4 is known to be activated by oxidants, heat, chemical and mechanical forces, and nutrient deprivation [6]. Lack of Klf4 induction can be associated with stress [70] and the Klf4-deficient lung of the Klf4 knockout mouse at birth exhibited signs of stress such as increased degree of apoptosis and p53 expression and dramatic induction of $p21^{CIP1//Waf1}$ independent of Klf4. The full implications of Klf4 expression in the perinatal period will require further study in vitro using Klf4 deficient and sufficient cell cultures and tissue explants, but ultimate proof will require a fibroblast-specific conditional deletion of Klf4 in vivo [71, 72]. But our study was the first to draw attention to a physiologic role for oxygen as a regulator of this transcription factor for fibroblast and myofibroblast differentiation in normal postnatal lung development [55]. The role of Klf4 in regulating these fibroblast populations during lung development is likely to be recapitulated in the adult lung during repair of lung injury and to involve interactions with other Kruppel-like family members. The newborn lung at birth could provide a window into the responsiveness of an organism to changes in the environment of oxygen and oxidant stress.

4. Glutathione in perinatal lung antioxidant defense and macrophage function

In the alveolar space, alveolar macrophage (AM) surveillance is the first line of defense in the immune response as they ingest and clear pathogens, release cytokines and chemokines to recruit other immune cells, serve as antigen presenting cells, and interact with other alveolar cells to fine-tune the immune response. In order to fulfill their roles as sensors, transmitters, and responders to inflammation, AMs respond to endogenous and exogenous danger signals by changing their repertoire of surface receptor expression and functional phenotype to promote either host defense, wound healing, or immune regulation. This plasticity in their biological responses, including differentiation, phenotype, immune functions, and cellular interactions, is determined in large part by their extracellular milieu [73]. However, the phenotype is not permanent and pathogens or changes in the underlying microenvironment can promote a change between a predominance of one set of characteristics to another phenotype. Depending on the different stimuli within the microenvironment within the alveolar space, alveolar macrophages are activated via distinct pathways that produce opposing effects on macrophage receptor expression, cytokine expression, and phagocytic function [74]. In response to interferon-γ (IFN-γ) or microbial products, macrophages become classically activated (M1) macrophages and produce inflammatory cytokines and reactive intermediates of oxygen and nitrogen. In response to interleukin-4 or -13, macrophages become alternatively activated (M2) and produce anti-inflammatory mediators such as the interleukin-1 receptor antagonist and TGF-β, promote tissue repair and remodeling, and become tolerant to stimulation by endotoxin in order to protect against overwhelming systemic inflammation. However, this immunosuppression is associated with a decreased capacity to clear microbes, and many diseases have abnormal shifts in the AM phenotype and immune responses that limit the ability of the cells to become innate immune effectors. Whether newborn AMs are skewed toward a M1 or M2 phenotype is unclear, but studies in a mouse model suggest that AM maturation in the fetal lung may include features of both pro-inflammatory and alternative activation paradigms [75].

Newborn infants, particularly those born preterm, face immunological challenges after birth because of the developmental stage of their immune systems. Upon birth, there is an age-dependent maturation of the intrapulmonary inflammatory responses with decreased AM immune responses such as phagocytosis and secretion of inflammatory mediators with potential immunoregulatory consequences [76, 77]. The functionally immature status of the newborn AM is suggested to be critical in the recurrent problem of early infancy pulmonary infections and morbidity [78]. At day 3 of life for premature newborns, the alveolar cells are more likely to have greater numbers of mononuclear phagocytes in the airway but fewer of these cells are functionally mature AMs [79]. This suggests that newborn AMs are functionally immature which may lead to increased susceptibility to lung infections. Furthermore, the degree of postnatal immune-suppression correlates with gestational age and is a predisposing factor for late infections [80].

The growth factor GM-CSF, granulocyte-macrophage colony stimulating factor, and its transcription factors PU.1 and Bach2 are increased after birth and necessary for AM differentiation and homeostasis making them critical to the AM immune response [81]. In newborn mice, the pleotropic peroxisome proliferator-activated receptor-γ (PPARγ) modulates several transcription factors and genes associated with AM differentiation and immune functions. However, PPARγ expression in fetal lung monocytes is dependent on the GM-CSF pathway suggesting that GM-CSF has a lung-specific role in the perinatal development of AMs through the induction of PPARγ in fetal monocytes. Therefore, factors that suppress GM-CSF or PPARγ expression in the newborn AM also suppress differentiation and the development of a mature immune response as summarized I recent reviews [82–85].

In *in vivo* studies, ROS induces upregulation of TGF-β expression [86], which is also a characteristic of a M2 phenotype [74]. Once TGF-β is activated, it induces the GSH depletion and increases intracellular ROS production. Children with severe asthma have significantly higher concentration of TGF-β in the epithelial lining fluid, which is associated with increased TGF-β and increased oxidative stress in the AMs [87]. In a mouse model, intranasal instillation of an adenovirus expressing constitutively active TGF-β results in suppression of the expression of both catalytic and modifier subunits of glutamate-cysteine ligase (GCL), the rate-limiting enzyme in de novo glutathione synthesis, decreased glutathione concentration, and increased protein and lipid peroxidation in mouse lung [88]. Similarly, M2 macrophages have robust increases in TGF-β1 production and secretion [74], thereby creating a vicious cycle of ROS generation, TGF-β production and signaling, and a M2 phenotype [89]. Indeed, mounting evidence suggests that AMs, particularly M2 AMs, are the predominant source of TGF-β in lung fibrosis and depleting M2-polarized macrophages during the progressive phase of fibrosis reduces TGF-β and collagen deposition [90]. In contrast, glutathione precursors induce proteolysis of the TGF-β type II receptor and disintegration of TGF-β1 [86]. Therefore, perturbations in glutathione availability and its redox status in the epithelial lining fluid are important modulators of the AM phenotype and immune functions.

In addition a role for gestational development in the AM phenotype and immune response, the role of fetal exposures and subsequent changes in the microenvironment on the AM phenotype must also be considered. In animal models, *in utero* ethanol exposure also promotes oxidant stress in the newborn lung as evidenced by decreased concentrations of the reduced moiety and increased concentration of the oxidized glutathione moiety in the alveolus and neonatal AM [91]. This oxidation of the glutathione redox state in the alveolar space was associated with increased expression of TGF-β and markers of a M2 phenotype in the newborn AM [92–94]. Impaired AM phagocytosis decreased the neonatal lung's defense against experimental Group B Strep as well as systemic sepsis [92]. However, addition of the glutathione precursor S-adenosyl-methionine (SAM-e) to the dam's diet restored the AM immune responses as well as decreased the experimental Group B Strep pneumonia and systemic sepsis in the newborn with fetal ethanol exposure. A central role for glutathione availability in the alveolar space in the AM immune functions was further supported by the ability of intranasal delivery of glutathione in the newborn to reverse the immune dysfunction associated with fetal ethanol exposure. These studies highlight the vital importance of glutathione availability in the alveolar space for AM immune functions and the neonatal lung's defense against bacterial infection [92].

Studies in the adult of chronic ethanol ingestion highlight the role of the glutathione redox state and oxidative stress in AM expression of TGF-β, GM-CSF/PU.1 signaling, PPARγ expression, immune functions, and risk of experimental pneumonia [89, 95–98]. In addition to GM-CSF, expression and activity of PU.1 are also dependent on Nrf2 and the antioxidant response element which are downregulated by alcohol-induced oxidant stress [99]. Alcohol exposure also upregulates KLF4 in AMs and treatments with GM-CSF or TGF-β enhance or dampen KLF4 expression and binding, respectively [100]. Treatment with siRNA against KLF4 normalizes the effects on expression of GM-CSF and TGF-β as well as AM immune functions. A potential dynamic interactive role for chronic oxidant stress on TGF-β, GM-CSF, PU.1, Nrf2, and KLF4 on the newborn AM phenotype and immune functions remains to be determined.

The most common form of newborn chronic lung disease, bronchopulmonary dysplasia (BPD), is thought to be caused by oxidative disruption of lung morphogenesis. Following birth,

http://dx.doi.org/10.5772/63819

various risk factors, including pulmonary or systemic infections, high concentrations of oxygen inspiration, and mechanical ventilation, may act synergistically, amplifying the inflammation. At birth, premature newborns have significantly lower glutathione concentrations than term newborns, and the lowest glutathione levels are associated with the infants with the most severe airways problems and required high oxygen support [101–104]. In intubated newborns, exhaled breath condensate samples correlated with tracheal aspirate samples in terms of reduced, oxidized, and total glutathione (GSH + GSSG) [105]. Decreased glutathione and subsequent oxidative stress in this microenvironment of the lining fluid was also observed in the AMs obtained from the tracheal aspirate. This glutathione deficiency and oxidative stress associated with the immature lung are likely to promote changes in the AM phenotype and immune functions, thereby increasing the risk of infection. This increased oxidative stress may contribute to the significant increased expression of TGF-β in the AMs of premature newborns [106, 107]. Further research is needed to specifically decipher the unique and complex mechanisms underlying AM maturation and pulmonary immune regulation at baseline and in response to oxidative stress. Pulmonary immune regulation in the premature neonate may be similar to the adult or it may be dramatically different because of the immaturity of the immune system.

5. Is birth an integrator that balances oxidant stress and antioxidant defense?

We have presented our work and ideas about the lung at birth and its experience of a major change in the oxygen environment. Clearly antioxidant gene induction is part of the developmental program in the late fetal lung and provides protection against oxidant stress. Other antioxidant genes are induced at birth in response to oxidant stress as an added source of protection. These activities are essential to a cell like the alveolar macrophage which must now populate the gas-filled alveolar space, protect against inhaled pathogens, and regulate

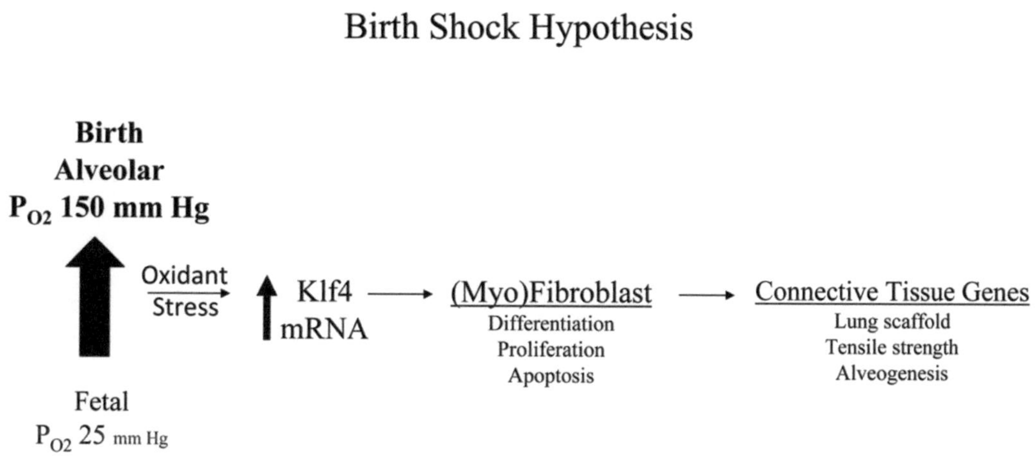

surfactant homeostasis. Nonetheless, the normal lung does not buffer all the oxidant stress it encounters at birth. Rather a transient but measurable degree of oxidant stress persists and we propose that this level serves a physiological function in our **birth shock hypothesis**. As the local redox state of lung cells changes, this signals the lung to initiate an alternative course for postnatal lung development. It is in effect a **"natural experiment with hyperoxia"** as the lung cannot predict the magnitude of the change in the oxygen environment that will ensue. It survives by balancing a level of redox stress that limits lung injury, while permitting activation of genes required for postnatal lung development. Birth then may serve as an integrator of these two competing ends. Our observations about the transcription factor Klf4 (**a birth shock protein**), fibroblast and myofibroblast and macrophage cell populations and the transcriptional regulators we described affecting cell proliferation, cell differentiation, and cell apoptosis in our studies are likely only the beginning of understanding this hypothesis. We believe that study of an event such as this in the newborn lung may provide new insight and strategies to assess, support, and manipulate the oxygen environment and oxidant stress to enable a more normal development for the premature lung at birth and repair of oxidant-induced injury in the developing and the mature lung.

Acknowledgements

Dr. Joyce-Brady was funded by NHLBI PO1 HL47049 and an Ignition Award from Boston University Office of Technology Development. Dr. Brown is funded by National Institutes on Alcohol Abuse and Alcoholism P50 AA-135757 and National Heart Lung And Blood Institute 1RO1 HL 125042 and 5R34 HL 117351.

Author details

Jyh-Chang Jean[1], Lou Ann Scism Brown[2] and Martin Joyce-Brady[1*]

*Address all correspondence to: mjbrady@bu.edu

1 The Pulmonary Center at Boston University School of Medicine, Boston, MA, USA

2 Department of Pediatrics, Emory University School of Medicine, Atlanta, GA, USA

References

[1] Muglia L, Jacobson L, Dikkes P, Majzoub JA. Corticotropin-releasing hormone deficiency reveals major fetal but not adult glucocorticoid need. Nature 1995;373:427–32.

[2] Joyce-Brady MF, Brody JS. Ontogeny of pulmonary alveolar epithelial markers of differentiation. Dev Biol 1990;137:331–48.

[3] Treutlein B, Brownfield DG, Wu AR, Neff NF, Mantalas GL, Espinoza FH, et al. Reconstructing lineage hierarchies of the distal lung epithelium using single-cell RNA-seq. Nature 2014 May 15;509(7500):371–5.

[4] Maeda Y, Dave V, Whitsett JA. Transcriptional control of lung morphogenesis. Physiol Rev 2007 Jan;87(1):219–44.

[5] St JD, Nusslein-Volhard C. The origin of pattern and polarity in the Drosophila embryo. Cell 1992 Jan 24;68(2):201–19.

[6] McConnell BB, Yang VW. Mammalian Kruppel-like factors in health and diseases. Physiol Rev 2010 Oct;90(4):1337–81.

[7] Wani MA, Wert SE, Lingrel JB. Lung Kruppel-like factor, a zinc finger transcription factor, is essential for normal lung development. J Biol Chem 1999 Jul 23;274(30):21180–5.

[8] Wan H, Luo F, Wert SE, Zhang L, Xu Y, Ikegami M, et al. Kruppel-like factor 5 is required for perinatal lung morphogenesis and function. Development 2008 Aug; 135(15):2563–72.

[9] Bieker JJ. Kruppel-like factors: three fingers in many pies. J Biol Chem 2001 Sep 14;276(37):34355–8.

[10] Brody JS, Thurlbeck W. Development, growth, and aging of the lung. Handbook of Physiology. The Respiratory System. Bethesda: American Physiological Society; 1986. p. 355–86.

[11] Kauffman SL, Burri PH, Weibel ER. The postnatal growth of the rat lung. II. Autoradiography. Anat Rec 1974 Sep;180(1):63–76.

[12] Adamson IY, King GM. Epithelial-mesenchymal interactions in postnatal rat lung growth. Exp Lung Res 1985;8(4):261–74.

[13] O'Hare KH, Townes PL. Morphogenesis of albino rat lung: an autoradiographic analysis of the embryological origin of the type I and II pulmonary epithelial cells. J Morphol 1970;132(1):69–87.

[14] Burri PH. The postnatal growth of the rat lung. 3. Morphology. Anat Rec 1974 Sep; 180(1):77–98.

[15] Vaccaro C, Brody JS. Ultrastructure of developing alveoli. Anat Rec 1978;192:467–80.

[16] Weinstein M, Xu X, Ohyama K, Deng CX. FGFR-3 and FGFR-4 function cooperatively to direct alveogenesis in the murine lung. Development 1998 Sep;125(18):3615–23.

[17] Bostrom H, Willetts K, Pekny M, Leveen P, Lindahl P, Hedstrand H, et al. PDGF-A signaling is a critical event in lung alveolar myofibroblast development and alveogenesis. Cell 1996 Jun 14;85(6):863–73.

[18] Nakamura T, Lozano PR, Ikeda Y, Iwanaga Y, Hinek A, Minamisawa S, et al. Fibulin-5/DANCE is essential for elastogenesis in vivo. Nature 2002 Jan 10;415(6868):171–5.

[19] Yanagisawa H, Davis EC, Starcher BC, Ouchi T, Yanagisawa M, Richardson JA, et al. Fibulin-5 is an elastin-binding protein essential for elastic fibre development in vivo. Nature 2002 Jan 10;415(6868):168–71.

[20] Chen H, Sun J, Buckley S, Chen C, Warburton D, Wang XF, et al. Abnormal mouse lung alveolarization caused by Smad3 deficiency is a developmental antecedent of centrilobular emphysema. Am J Physiol Lung Cell Mol Physiol 2005 Apr;288(4):L683–L691.

[21] Morris DG, Huang X, Kaminski N, Wang Y, Shapiro SD, Dolganov G, et al. Loss of integrin alpha(v)beta6-mediated TGF-beta activation causes Mmp12-dependent emphysema. Nature 2003 Mar 13;422(6928):169–73.

[22] Rishikof DC, Lucey EC, Kuang PP, Snider GL, Goldstein RH. Induction of the myofibroblast phenotype following elastolytic injury to mouse lung. Histochem Cell Biol 2006 May;125(5):527–34.

[23] Nardell EA, Brody JS. Determinants of mechanical properties of rat lung during postnatal development. J Appl Physiol 1982 Jul;53(1):140–8.

[24] Kaczynski J, Cook T, Urrutia R. Sp1-and Kruppel-like transcription factors. Genome Biology 2003;4(2):206.

[25] Mahatan C, Kaestner K, Geiman D, Yang V. Characterization of the structure and regulation of the murine gene encoding gut-enriched Kruppel-like factor (Kruppel-like factor 4). Nuc Acids Res 1999;27(23):4562–9.

[26] Lomberk G, Urrutia R. The family feud: turning off Sp1 by Sp1-like KLF proteins. Biochemical Journal 2005 Nov 15;392:1–11.

[27] Philipsen S, Suske G. A tale of three fingers: the family of mammalian Sp/XKLF transcription factors. Nucleic Acids Res 1999 Aug 1;27(15):2991–3000.

[28] Wei D, Kanai M, Huang S, Xie K. Emerging role of KLF4 in human gastrointestinal cancer. Carcinogenesis 2006 Jan;27(1):23–31.

[29] Mariani TJ, Reed JJ, Shapiro SD. Expression profiling of the developing mouse lung: Insights into the establishment of the extracellular matrix. Am J Respir Cell Mol Biol 2002;26:541–8.

[30] Wani MA, Wert SE, Lingrel JB. Lung Kruppel-like factor, a zinc finger transcription factor, is essential for normal lung development. J Biol Chem 1999 Jul 23;274(30):21180–5.

[31] Garrett-Sinha L, Eberspaecher H, Seldin M, de Crombrugghe B. A gene for a novel zinc-finger protein expressed in differentiated epithelial cells and transiently in certain mesenchymal cells. J Biol Chem 1996;271:31384–90.

[32] Shields J, Christy R, Yang V. Identification and characterization of a gene encoding a gut-enriched Kruppel-like factor expressed during growth arrest. J Biol Chem 1996;271(33):20009–17.

[33] Ohnishi KTMKYSSKYT. Matrix metalloproteinase-mediated extracellular matrix protein degradation in human pulmonary emphysema. Lab Invest 1998;78(9):1077–87.

[34] Laub F, Aldabe R, Ramirez F, Friedman S. Embryonic expression of Kruppel-like factor 6 in neural and non-neural tissues. Mechanisms of Development 2001 Aug;106(1–2): 167–70.

[35] Imataka H, Sogawa K, Yasumoto K, Kikuchi Y, Sasano K, Kobayashi A, et al. Two regulatory proteins that bind to the basic transcription element (BTE), a GC box sequence in the promoter region of the rat P-4501A1 gene. EMBO J 1992 Oct;11(10): 3663–71.

[36] Scohy S, Gabant P, Van RT, Hertveldt V, Dreze PL, Van VP, et al. Identification of KLF13 and KLF14 (SP6), novel members of the SP/XKLF transcription factor family. Genomics 2000 Nov 15;70(1):93–101.

[37] Chiambaretta F, De GF, Turet G, Marceau G, Gain P, Dastugue B, et al. Cell and tissue specific expression of human Kruppel-like transcription factors in human ocular surface. Mol Vis 2004 Nov 23;10:901–9.

[38] Zhang W, Geiman DE, Shields JM, Dang DT, Mahatan CS, Kaestner KH, et al. The gut-enriched Kruppel-like factor (Kruppel-like factor 4) mediates the transactivating effect of p53 on the $p21^{WAF1/Cip1}$ promoter. J Biol Chem 2000 Jun 16;275(24):18391–8.

[39] Dang DT, Bachman KE, Mahatan CS, Dang LH, Giardiello FM, Yang VW. Decreased expression of the gut-enriched Kruppel-like factor gene in intestinal adenomas of multiple intestinal neoplasia mice and in colonic adenomas of familial adenomatous polyposis patients. FEBS Lett 2000 Jul 7;476(3):203–7.

[40] Ton-That H, Kaestner KH, Shields JM, Mahatanankoon CS, Yang VW. Expression of the gut-enriched Kruppel-like factor gene during development and intestinal tumorigenesis. FEBS Lett 1997 Dec 15;419(2–3):239–43.

[41] Dang DT, Mahatan CS, Dang LH, Agboola IA, Yang VW. Expression of the gut-enriched Kruppel-like factor (Kruppel-like factor 4) gene in the human colon cancer cell line RKO is dependent on CDX2. Oncogene 2001 Aug 9;20(35):4884–90.

[42] Chen X, Whitney EM, Gao SY, Yang VW. Transcriptional profiling of Kruppel-like factor 4 reveals a function in cell cycle regulation and epithelial differentiation. J Mol Biol 2003 Feb 21;326(3):665–77.

[43] Shie JL, Chen ZY, Fu M, Pestell RG, Tseng CC. Gut-enriched Kruppel-like factor represses cyclin D1 promoter activity through Sp1 motif. Nucleic Acids Res 2000 Aug 1;28(15):2969–76.

[44] Segre J, Bauer C, Fuchs E. Klf4 is a transcription factor required for establishing the barrier function of the skin. Nature Genetics 1999;22(4):356–60.

[45] Katz J, Perreault N, Goldstein B, Lee C, Labosky P, Yang V, et al. The zinc-finger transcription factor Klf4 is required for terminal differentiation of goblet cells in the colon. Development 2002;129(11):2619–28.

[46] Yet SF, McA'Nulty MM, Folta SC, Yen HW, Yoshizumi M, Hsieh CM, et al. Human EZF, a Kruppel-like zinc finger protein, is expressed in vascular endothelial cells and contains transcriptional activation and repression domains. J Biol Chem 1998 Jan 9;273(2):1026–31.

[47] Peters DG, Zhang XC, Benos PV, Heidrich-O'Hare E, Ferrell RE. Genomic analysis of immediate/early response to shear stress in human coronary artery endothelial cells. Physiol Genomics 2002 Dec 26;12(1):25–33.

[48] Roy S, Khanna S, Wallace WA, Lappalainen J, Rink C, Cardounel AJ, et al. Characterization of perceived hyperoxia in isolated primary cardiac fibroblasts and in the reoxygenated heart. J Biol Chem 2003 Nov 21;278(47):47129–35.

[49] Nickenig G, Baudler S, Muller C, Werner C, Werner N, Welzel H, et al. Redox-sensitive vascular smooth muscle cell proliferation is mediated by GKLF and Id3 in vitro and in vivo. FASEB J 2002 Jul;16(9):1077–86.

[50] Bonner ALWYM. Gene expression signatures identify novel regulatory pathways during murine lung development: implications for lung tumorigenesis. J Medical Genetics 2003;40:408–17.

[51] Landesberg L, Ramalingam R, Lee K, Rosengart T, Crystal R. Upregulation of transcription factors in lung in the early phase of postpneumonectomy lung growth. Amer J Physiol Lung Cell Mol Physiol 2001;281:L1138–L1149.

[52] Spira A, Beane J, Shah V, Liu G, Schembri F, Yang X, et al. Effects of cigarette smoke on the human airway epithelial cell transcriptome. Proc Natl Acad Sci USA 2004 Jul 6;101(27):10143–8.

[53] Wang J, Wang S, Manzer R, McConville G, Mason RJ. Ozone induces oxidative stress in rat alveolar type II and type I-like cells. Free Radic Biol Med 2006 Jun 1;40(11):1914–28.

[54] Hu B, Wu Z, Liu T, Ullenbruch MR, Jin H, Phan SH. Gut-enriched Kruppel-like factor interaction with Smad3 inhibits myofibroblast differentiation. Am J Respir Cell Mol Biol 2006 Jul 20. 2007;36(1);78–84.

[55] Jean JC, George E, Kaestner KH, Brown LA, Spira A, Joyce-Brady M. Transcription factor Klf4, induced in the lung by oxygen at birth, regulates perinatal fibroblast and myofibroblast differentiation. PLoS One 2013;8(1):e54806.

[56] Chen Y, Frank L. Differential gene expression of antioxidant enzymes in the perinatal rat lung. Pediatric Research 1993;34:27–31.

[57] Das KC, Guo X-L, White CW. Induction of thioredoxin and thioredoxin reductase gene expression in lungs of newborn primates by oxygen. Am J Physiol 1999;276:530–9.

[58] Das KC, Phl PMB, Guo X, White CW. Induction of Peroxiredoxin Gene Expression by Oxygen In Lungs of Newborn Primates. Am J Respir Cell Mol Biol 2001;In press.

[59] Land SC, Wilson SM. Redox regulation of lung development and perinatal lung epithelial function. Antioxid Redox Signal 2005;7(1–2):92–107.

[60] Chen X, Johns D, Geiman D, Marban E, Dang D, Hamlin G, et al. Kruppel-like factor 4 (gut-enriched Kruppel-like factor) inhibits cell proliferation by blocking G1/S progression of the cell cycle. J Biol Chem 2001;276(32):30423–8.

[61] Nardell EA, Brody JS. Determinants of mechanical properties of rat lung during postnatal development. J Appl Physiol Respir Environ Exerc Physiol 1982 Jul;53(1):140–8.

[62] Foronjy R, D'Armiento J. The role of collagenase in emphysema. Respir Res 2001;2(6): 348–52.

[63] Hinz B, Gabbiani G. Cell-matrix and cell-cell contacts of myofibroblasts: role in connective tissue remodeling. Thromb Haemost 2003 Dec;90(6):993–1002.

[64] Lindahl P, Karlsson L, Hellstrom M, Gebre-Medhin S, Willetts K, Heath JK, et al. Alveogenesis failure in PDGF-A-deficient mice is coupled to lack of distal spreading of alveolar smooth muscle cell progenitors during lung development. Development 1997 Oct;124(20):3943–53.

[65] McGowan SE. Extracellular matrix and the regulation of lung development and repair. FASEB J 1992;6:2895–904.

[66] Wagner TE, Frevert CW, Herzog EL, Schnapp LM. Expression of the integrin subunit alpha8 in murine lung development. J Histochem Cytochem 2003 Oct;51(10):1307–15.

[67] Liu Y, Sinha S, McDonald OG, Shang Y, Hoofnagle MH, Owens GK. Kruppel-like factor 4 abrogates myocardin-induced activation of smooth muscle gene expression. J Biol Chem 2005 Mar 11;280(10):9719–27.

[68] Scavo LM, Ertsey R, Chapin CJ, Allen L, Kitterman JA. Apoptosis in the development of rat and human fetal lungs. Am J Respir Cell Mol Biol 1998 Jan;18(1):21–31.

[69] Schittny JC, Djonov V, Fine A, Burri P. Programmed Cell Death Contributes to Postnatal Lung Development. Amer J Respir Cell Mol Biol 1998;18:786–93.

[70] Toledano MB. The guardian recruits cops: the p53-p21 axis delegates prosurvival duties to the Keap1-Nrf2 stress pathway. Mol Cell 2009 Jun 26;34(6):637–9.

[71] Katz JP, Perreault N, Goldstein BG, Actman L, McNally SR, Silberg DG, et al. Loss of Klf4 in mice causes altered proliferation and differentiation and precancerous changes in the adult stomach. Gastroenterology 2005 Apr;128(4):935–45.

[72] Swamynathan SK, Katz JP, Kaestner KH, Ashery-Padan R, Crawford MA, Piatigorsky J. Conditional deletion of the mouse Klf4 gene results in corneal epithelial fragility, stromal edema, and loss of conjunctival goblet cells. Mol Cell Biol 2007 Jan;27(1):182–94.

[73] Aggarwal NR, King LS, D'Alessio FR. Diverse macrophage populations mediate acute lung inflammation and resolution. Am J Physiol Lung Cell Mol Physiol 2014 Apr 15;306(8):L709–L725.

[74] Martinez FO, Gordon S. The M1 and M2 paradigm of macrophage activation: time for reassessment. F1000Prime Rep 2014;6:13.

[75] Stouch AN, Zaynagetdinov R, Barham WJ, Stinnett AM, Slaughter JC, Yull FE, et al. IkappaB kinase activity drives fetal lung macrophage maturation along a non-M1/M2 paradigm. J Immunol 2014 Aug 1;193(3):1184–93.

[76] Islam MA, Uddin MJ, Tholen E, Tesfaye D, Looft C, Schellander K, et al. Age-related changes in phagocytic activity and production of pro-inflammatory cytokines by lipopolysaccharide stimulated porcine alveolar macrophages. CYTOKINE 2012 Dec; 60(3):707–17.

[77] Kurkjian C, Hollifield M, Lines JL, Rogosky A, Empey KM, Qureshi M, et al. Alveolar macrophages in neonatal mice are inherently unresponsive to Pneumocystis murina infection. Infect Immun 2012 Aug;80(8):2835–46.

[78] Martin TR, Ruzinski JT, Wilson CB, Skerrett SJ. Effects of endotoxin in the lungs of neonatal rats: age-dependent impairment of the inflammatory response. J Infect Dis 1995 Jan;171(1):134–44.

[79] Prince LR, Maxwell NC, Gill SK, Dockrell DH, Sabroe I, McGreal EP, et al. Macrophage phenotype is associated with disease severity in preterm infants with chronic lung disease. PLoS One 2014;9(8):e103059.

[80] Palojarvi A, Petaja J, Siitonen S, Janer C, Andersson S. Low monocyte HLA-DR expression as an indicator of immunodepression in very low birth weight infants. Pediatr Res 2013 Apr;73(4 Pt 1):469–75.

[81] Iwabuchi H, Kawasaki T, Yamamoto T, Uchiyama M, Nakata K, Naito M. Expression of PU.1 and terminal differentiation of alveolar macrophages in newborn rats. Cell Tissue Res 2007 Jul;329(1):71–9.

[82] Divangahi M, King IL, Pernet E. Alveolar macrophages and type I IFN in airway homeostasis and immunity. Trends Immunol 2015 May;36(5):307–14.

[83] Hussell T, Bell TJ. Alveolar macrophages: plasticity in a tissue-specific context. Nat Rev Immunol 2014 Feb;14(2):81–93.

[84] Morales-Nebreda L, Misharin AV, Perlman H, Budinger GR. The heterogeneity of lung macrophages in the susceptibility to disease. Eur Respir Rev 2015 Sep;24(137):505–9.

[85] Schneider C, Nobs SP, Kurrer M, Rehrauer H, Thiele C, Kopf M. Induction of the nuclear receptor PPAR-gamma by the cytokine GM-CSF is critical for the differentiation of fetal monocytes into alveolar macrophages. Nat Immunol 2014 Nov;15(11):1026–37.

[86] Koli K, Myllarniemi M, Keski-Oja J, Kinnula VL. Transforming growth factor-beta activation in the lung: focus on fibrosis and reactive oxygen species. Antioxid Redox Signal 2008 Feb;10(2):333–42.

[87] Brown SD, Baxter KM, Stephenson ST, Esper AM, Brown LA, Fitzpatrick AM. Airway TGF-beta1 and oxidant stress in children with severe asthma: association with airflow limitation. J Allergy Clin Immunol 2012 Feb;129(2):388–96, 396.

[88] Liu RM, Vayalil PK, Ballinger C, Dickinson DA, Huang WT, Wang S, et al. Transforming growth factor beta suppresses glutamate-cysteine ligase gene expression and induces oxidative stress in a lung fibrosis model. Free Radic Biol Med 2012 Aug 1;53(3):554–63.

[89] Brown SD, Brown LA. Ethanol (EtOH)-induced TGF-beta1 and reactive oxygen species production are necessary for EtOH-induced alveolar macrophage dysfunction and induction of alternative activation. Alcohol Clin Exp Res 2012 Nov;36(11):1952–62.

[90] Murthy S, Larson-Casey JL, Ryan AJ, He C, Kobzik L, Carter AB. Alternative activation of macrophages and pulmonary fibrosis are modulated by scavenger receptor, macrophage receptor with collagenous structure. FASEB J 2015 Aug;29(8):3527–36.

[91] Ping XD, Harris FL, Brown LA, Gauthier TW. In vivo dysfunction of the term alveolar macrophage after in utero ethanol exposure. Alcohol Clin Exp Res 2007 Feb;31(2):308–16.

[92] Gauthier TW, Young PA, Gabelaia L, Tang SM, Ping XD, Harris FL, et al. In utero ethanol exposure impairs defenses against experimental group B streptococcus in the term Guinea pig lung. Alcohol Clin Exp Res 2009 Feb;33(2):300–6.

[93] Gauthier TW, Ping XD, Gabelaia L, Brown LA. Delayed neonatal lung macrophage differentiation in a mouse model of in utero ethanol exposure. Am J Physiol Lung Cell Mol Physiol 2010 Jul;299(1):L8–16.

[94] Konomi JV, Harris FL, Ping XD, Gauthier TW, Brown LA. Zinc insufficiency mediates ethanol-induced alveolar macrophage dysfunction in the pregnant female mouse. Alcohol Alcohol 2015 Jan;50(1):30–8.

[95] Joshi PC, Applewhite L, Ritzenthaler JD, Roman J, Fernandez AL, Eaton DC, et al. Chronic ethanol ingestion in rats decreases granulocyte-macrophage colony-stimulat-

ing factor receptor expression and downstream signaling in the alveolar macrophage. J Immunol 2005 Nov 15;175(10):6837–45.

[96] Yeligar SM, Harris FL, Hart CM, Brown LA. Ethanol induces oxidative stress in alveolar macrophages via upregulation of NADPH oxidases. J Immunol 2012 Apr 15;188(8): 3648–57.

[97] Yeligar SM, Harris FL, Hart CM, Brown LA. Glutathione attenuates ethanol-induced alveolar macrophage oxidative stress and dysfunction by downregulating NADPH oxidases. Am J Physiol Lung Cell Mol Physiol 2014 Mar 1;306(5):L429–L441.

[98] Yeligar SM, Mehta AJ, Harris FL, Brown LA, Hart CM. PPARgamma regulates chronic alcohol-induced alveolar macrophage dysfunction. Am J Respir Cell Mol Biol 2015 Dec 17. 2015 Dec17-DOI 10.1165/rcmb.2015-0077OC.

[99] Staitieh BS, Egea EE, Fan X, Azih N, Neveu W, Guidot DM. Activation of alveolar macrophages with interferon-gamma promotes antioxidant defenses via the Nrf2-ARE pathway. J Clin Cell Immunol 2015 Oct;6(5).

[100] Curry-McCoy TV, Guidot DM, Joshi PC. Chronic alcohol ingestion in rats decreases Kruppel-like factor 4 expression and intracellular zinc in the lung. Alcohol Clin Exp Res 2013 Mar;37(3):361–71.

[101] Collard KJ, Godeck S, Holley JE, Quinn MW. Pulmonary antioxidant concentrations and oxidative damage in ventilated premature babies. Arch Dis Child Fetal Neonatal Ed 2004 Sep;89(5):F412–F416.

[102] Grigg J, Barber A, Silverman M. Bronchoalveolar lavage fluid glutathione in intubated premature infants. Arch Dis Child 1993 Jul;69(1 Spec No):49–51.

[103] Jain A, Mehta T, Auld PA, Rodrigues J, Ward RF, Schwartz MK, et al. Glutathione metabolism in newborns: evidence for glutathione deficiency in plasma, bronchoalveolar lavage fluid, and lymphocytes in prematures. Pediatr Pulmonol 1995 Sep;20(3): 160–6.

[104] Reise JA, Taylor GW, Fardy CH, Silverman M. Glutathione and neonatal lung disease. Clin Chim Acta 1997 Sep 8;265(1):113–9.

[105] Rosso MI, Roark S, Taylor E, Ping X, Ward JM, Roche K, et al. Exhaled breath condensate in intubated neonates—a window into the lung's glutathione status. Respir Res 2014;15:1.

[106] Kwong KY, Niang S, Literat A, Zhu NL, Ramanathan R, Jones CA, et al. Expression of transforming growth factor beta (TGF-b1) by human preterm lung inflammatory cells. Life Sci 2006 Nov 17;79(25):2349–56.

[107] Strandjord TP, Clark JG, Guralnick DE, Madtes DK. Immunolocalization of transforming growth factor-alpha, epidermal growth factor (EGF), and EGF-receptor in normal and injured developing human lung. Pediatr Res 1995 Dec;38(6):851–6.

Chapter 9

Non-Pulmonary Management of Newborns with Respiratory Distress

Petja Fister and Štefan Grosek

Additional information is available at the end of the chapter

http://dx.doi.org/10.5772/63386

Abstract

Due to the developmental immaturity of the lungs and other organs, the premature newborns are more prone to develop respiratory distress syndrome (RDS) and other problems of prematurity. The prevention of heat and water loses improves survival. Intolerance to excessive fluids and electrolytes in the transitional period may affect urine and sodium excretion together with maladaptation of cardiovascular system, the development of heart failure, and deterioration of RDS due to patent ductus arteriosus (PDA) and further development of bronchopulmonary dysplasia (BPD). Closure of PDA is frequently needed. The "trophic feeding" and intensive nutrition as soon as possible prevent weight loss and further growth restriction. Greater sensitivity to pain, short- and long-term effects of inappropriately treated pain, use of opioids and sedatives are of concern in the short- and long-term outcomes. Cardiovascular stability and adequate perfusion of the brain both affect the neurological outcome. Delayed cord clamping and erythropoietin help maintaining adequate levels of circulating hemoglobin which might affect later cognitive outcomes. In the following sections, detailed descriptions of non-pulmonary management will be presented. We conducted electronic searches of articles on supportive (non-pulmonary) management of newborns with RDS. Consensus guidelines on newborns with respiratory distress have been reviewed.

Keywords: newborns, evidence-based therapy, antenatal steroids, transport in utero, regionalization of maternity hospitals and neonatal intensive care units, thermoregulation, fluid, nutrition, antibiotics, pain, blood pressure, perfusion, patent ductus arteriosus

1. Introduction

Non-pulmonary management of newborns with respiratory distress syndrome (RDS) is neither the last nor the least important part of the management, but it is supposed to be involved and intertwined in the whole necessary work-up integrated for the well-being of the tinny newborn. Each momentum from the prenatal care, pregnancy, and finally to the birth of the newborn should be considered when we are aiming to improve the final outcome, that is, delivery of a healthy newborn. Pulmonary management of newborns with RDS is only one, though very important and lifesaving, but not sufficient and adequate part of the whole care management of the newborns with RDS.

2. Methods

This chapter will look at the importance of prenatal care, temperature control, control of hypoglycemia, fluid and nutritional intake, the impact of perinatal infection and the use and misuse of antibiotics, frequency of unnecessary procedures, proper pain management, the impact of excessive use of opiates on ventilation duration in the management of newborns with RDS. The impact of optimal blood pressure, tissue perfusion, and patent ductus arteriosus (PDA) with hemodynamic management in newborns with RDS is going to be reviewed. Also, the short- and long-term outcomes in respect of supportive management of newborns in the intensive care unit will be addressed. We conducted electronic searches of articles on supportive (non-pulmonary) management and reviewed the consensus guidelines on management of newborns with RDS [1].

3. Prenatal care

Every newborn can develop RDS, but the likelihood among the premature infants to be affected with the RDS is the highest [2, 3]. Therefore, as neonatal RDS is a disease predominantly affecting the preterm newborns, all the measures to decrease preterm delivery encompass its management. Preconception advice starting in teenage youth to prevent pregnancy in too young teenage girls is important, and social programs should be developed and delivered among the youths. This is not only the problem in poor countries in the world but is even more problematic in wealthy countries with high-gross domestic product but also extreme social inequalities. This preconception advice is closely related to proper protection from the sexually transmitted diseases which may also affect the fetal and later newborn's life. Both, youth pregnancy and sexually transmitted diseases together with under- or malnutrition, strongly affect the development of the fetus and premature delivery. Publically available access to the proper maternity care, at least in well-developed countries, should be offered to every pregnant woman: adequate number of visits at the obstetrician's, appropriate number of obstetric ultrasounds, teaching programs and screening for infections, developmental malformations, etc. Special problems are unwanted pregnancies because any termination of unwanted pregnancy brings different problems to the mother and future wanted pregnancies, but it is worth mentioning that illegal and criminal or nonprofessional abortion endangers the health and lives of the women [4].

In well-organized health systems, ultrasound measurement of cervical length in midtrimester enables prediction of preterm labor and women with short cervix (<25 mm) should be offered vaginal progesterone treatment [5]. Women with threatening preterm labor should be transferred by "in utero" transport to tertiary level medical centers where better outcomes in regards to mothers and newborns can be provided [6]. In the case of preterm premature rupture of membranes (PPROM), after reassuring maternal and fetal wellbeing threatened preterm delivery can be delayed by antibiotics treatment for 7 days to mothers from about 23 weeks up to 34 weeks of gestation [7]. Antibiotics reduce the rate of chorioamnionitis, preterm birth, infection, and respiratory insufficiency [8]. On the contrary, antibiotics have not been proved beneficial for mothers with preterm labor and intact membranes [9]. Delaying the preterm delivery has been also proved for magnesium sulfate which also has beneficial effects for the brain of the preterm newborn [10]. Preterm labor is efficaciously postponed by tocolytics [11]. Antenatal steroids given to mothers from about 23 weeks up to 34 weeks of gestation decrease the risk of neonatal death, RDS, intraventricular hemorrhage (IVH), and necrotizing entero-colitis (NEC) [12]. Moreover, antenatal steroids given more than 24 h and <7 days before elective cesarean section at term also influence the RDS in the late-preterm or term newborn [13]. Until further studies are done, one repeated dose of antenatal steroids given a week after the first dose is recommended [14].

Chorioamnionitis describes intrauterine inflammation of maternal and fetal tissues and endangers both, the mother and the newborn. It has been recognized as the major risk factor for preterm birth, prematurity-associated mortality in morbidity of newborns: the neonatal sepsis, RDS, cystic periventricular leukomalacia (PVL), IVH, and cerebral palsy [15, 16]. Since guidelines for the prevention of perinatal group B streptococcal (GBS) disease have been published, the incidence of early-onset GBS disease in newborns has dramatically decreased. The mayor prevention key is universal antenatal GBS screening of pregnant women and intrapartum antibiotic prophylaxis (IAP) for women with high-risk of infection with penicillin, ampicillin, or cefazolin. Adequate IAP is achieved by infusion of antibiotics at least 4 h before delivery [17].

4. Interhospital, "in utero" transport, and regionalization

Interhospital air and ground transportation of critically ill neonates, regionalization, organization of "in utero" transportations, and new tertiary perinatal centers, which care for the most at risk premature newborns, have greatly decreased the perinatal mortality rate over the last 30 years all over the world [6]. As an example, we present the results from the Republic of Slovenia where we have greatly decreased the perinatal mortality rate over the last 30 years to a rate of 3.5% for neonates weighing at least 1000 g in 2006. We have organized transportation since 1976, and we have transport "in utero" in two Slovenian perinatal centers since 1985 [18].

5. Temperature management

From the neonatal history, we learned that misunderstanding the adverse effects of low body temperature in the premature infants was related to higher mortality rate in hypothermic infants. With understanding the importance of normal body temperature later together with the invention of heated air incubators, the mortality rate dropped as much as twice immediately [19–21]. After birth, the newborn baby is exposed to extrauterine environment with temperature changes in relation to the environmental temperatures which are usually lower than the body temperature. Newborns and especially preterms have increased proportion of body surface in relation to body volume, their body has low-temperature capacity, and their skin is immature with increased water permeability. They also have low supplies of skin fat. Since oxygen and energy consumption are lowest in the range of thermal neutrality, it is important to keep newborns in those limited ambient temperature ranges to enable them to have their body temperature ranging from 36.5 to 37.5°C. By acknowledging the importance of thermal neutrality, this is one of the most manageable problems of non-pulmonary management of newborns with RDS [22].

Temperature regulation enables optimal efficiency of the metabolic processes and enzyme activities with the lowest oxygen and calorie consumption. Newborns are unable to produce sufficient heat by metabolic reactions, by muscle activity during motion, and by nonshivering thermogenesis in the brown fat, which starts to evolve between 26th and 30th weeks of gestation. Loosing heath from the body is modulated by changing the vascular tone of peripheral vessels and by sweating, which is not fully developed by the 36th week of gestation.

There are four ways newborns may lose heat to the environment. Immediately after birth, they are wet from the amniotic fluid and evaporation decreases their body temperature fast so all the measures to dry their body have to be taken. Recently, to decrease evaporation from the immature water permeable skin, very premature newborns, still wet, are immediately wrapped into plastic wraps or bags and caps [23–27]. To lessen the evaporation, the air in the incubators for all the preterms beyond 31 weeks of gestation should be humidified (60–80%) and preterm newborns should not be bathed until they can maintain their body temperature. The humidity should be decreased by 5% every day if they can maintain stable body temperature, and stopped when preterms can maintain their body temperature in 40% humidity [28]. Every object radiates—it gives or receives the heat in relation to the temperature difference. Therefore, it is important to keep the air temperature in a defined range and also to take into account the external temperatures, the room walls and windows and the isolation walls of the incubators [29]. Objects can lose heat by losing or gaining heat from the object in contact by conduction. Placing the newborn baby to the mother's abdomen allows skin to skin contact besides parental bonding and enables conduction of the heat from the mother to the child [22, 30–32]. Resuscitation on wet basis can cause a huge heat loss from the newborn and should be avoided. Infusing cold fluids also causes conduction loss of heat. Moving air causes heat loss by convection.

Hypothermia may lead to hypoglycemia or acidosis and has been associated with increased mortality, increased risk of late-onset sepsis, IVH, pulmonary insufficiency, and hemorrhage

[20, 21]. The vicious cycle of cooling causes norepinephrine release with pulmonary and peripheral vasoconstriction with increased right-to-left shunting of blood and maintenance of fetal circulation postnatally. To enable thermal neutrality, preterm newborns should be nursed in preheated and humidified incubators, and in heated beds after 32nd week of gestation or >1500 g. We provide them heated and humidified gases and clothe newborns with clothes and caps [33, 34].

6. Perinatal infection management

After the initial care of the newborn in the delivery room with drying the newborn's skin, providing warmth, positioning the head, and clearing the airway, the evaluation of respiration, and consequently oxygenation of peripheral organs follows. In case transitional period is prolonged and the signs of RDS persist, we have to obtain chest radiograph, blood gas analysis and perform sepsis work-up with complete blood count and cultures and start empirical antibiotic treatment with ampicillin or penicillin and gentamicin, especially if risk factors for early-onset sepsis are present. Early-onset infection with GBS typically imitates the RDS in preterm newborns with the clinical presentation and also radiographically so usually it is difficult to differentiate pneumonia from RDS without infection. Besides GBS congenital pneumonia can be caused by *Escherichia coli* and other microorganisms [35]. A well appearing newborn to a mother with chorioamnionitis should have a limited diagnostic evaluation and receive empirical antibiotic therapy. Well-appearing term newborns, born to mothers with appropriate IAP or inappropriate IAP with rupture of membranes for <18 h, need routine care and observation. Those term newborns whose mothers had inappropriate IAP and rupture of membranes for more than 18 h and all preterm newborns with inadequate IAP need clinical and laboratory evaluation and observation [17, 36]. There is no evidence to support routine antibiotic treatment of newborns with RDS and without risk factors for early-onset sepsis [37, 38]. In those newborns with RDS which do not have laboratory signs of sepsis and have negative cultures, the antibiotics should be discontinued as early as feasible [37, 39].

Late-onset sepsis occurs in one-fifth of premature newborns and is associated with increased mortality, prolonged hospitalization, and prolonged artificial ventilation, PDA, NEC, and BPD [40]. Newborns that were treated for neonatal sepsis later are at risk of poor weight gain and adverse neurodevelopmental outcome [41].

7. Fluid and electrolyte management

After birth, water and electrolyte balance is influenced by transitional and developmental adaptations of the newborn. More preterm newborns have more total body water, and extracellular fluid volume constitutes a greater part of total body water in comparison with term newborns. Furthermore, after birth, renal function of preterm newborns is reduced in comparison with term newborns and they lose more weight with diuresis which results from an isotonic reduction of extracellular fluid. Newborns, especially more preterm ones loose water insensibly through the skin and respiratory system, especially in RDS, when respiratory rate is increased [42, 43]. Insensible water loss is increased by radiant heaters, phototherapeutic lights, and inappropriate water content of inspired air. Antenatal steroids besides the already mentioned effect on lung maturation also accelerate skin and kidney maturation. Preterm newborns whose mothers have received antenatal steroids had lower insensible water loss, less hypernatremia, earlier diuresis and natriuresis, and less nonoliguric hyperkalemia [44, 45]. In the first postnatal days, water balance is kept in a slightly negative state. Excessive fluid administration is associated with increased risk of PDA, NEC, and BPD [46]. Fluid balance and volume status can be evaluated by physical examination with signs of hydration, edema, and hemodynamic stability, body weight loss or gain, balance of fluid intake and output, and biochemistry evaluation of electrolyte concentration in plasma of the newborns. Fluid requirements therefore account for maintenance requirements, obligatory losses, and possible deficits and are gestational and postnatal age, ambient temperature and humidity, renal and respiratory function dependent. The electrolyte requirements for sodium, potassium, and chloride are approximately 1–2 mEq/kg/day except for the first day when isotonic reduction of extracellular fluid ensues. Diuretics cause electrolyte disturbances due to urinary loss of sodium and potassium and loop diuretics are associated with nephrocalcinosis so we prefer not to use them routinely [47].

8. Nutritional management

The newborn's nutritional status is influenced by his past history with genetic background, maternal body composition, and nutrition before and during pregnancy [48]. Many preterm newborns are born growth restricted because of inadequate intrauterine nutrient supply. Postnatal nutrition and metabolic capacity impact postnatal growth and development and have long-term consequences on the lung, brain, and other organ development and cognitive function [49]. The newborn's brain consumes half of all the energy provided, and too little calories mean less brain volume and worse neurocognitive outcome. Adequate volume of fluids, the protein content, and energy balance in the newborn's, and especially preterm's nutrition should cover metabolic expenditure and growth requirements, thus setting the ground for optimal outcomes.

In newborns with RDS, early enteral feeding is frequently delayed because of concomitant medical problems and fear of complications as the feeding intolerance and NEC. Therefore, the parenteral nutrition is commenced as early as possible to correct prenatal, to prevent postnatal growth failure and to improve outcomes [50, 51]. The parenteral nutrition has to provide enough calories for energy and growth, which are met by carbohydrates, proteins, and lipids. Carbohydrates provide glucose, proteins provide essential amino acids and nitrogen, and lipids provide essential fatty acids. Essential nutrients needed for growth are electrolytes, vitamins, minerals, and trace elements [52–54].

The premature newborn needs parenterally about 100 kcal/kg/day of nonprotein energy for growing, 3/5 in the form of carbohydrates and 2/5 in the form of lipids. Glucose is the form of carbohydrates that we give parenterally, and it is the primary energy supply for the newborn's brain. We start with 7 g/kg/day of glucose, which provides 4.8 mg/kg/min of glucose, and we increase the amount by 1.5–2 g/kg/day, up to 15 g/kg/day and maximum of 18 g/kg/day (12.5 mg/kg/min). Preterm newborns are prone to hypoglycemia because of higher glucose needs, decreased fat stores, and higher-energy consumption. On the other hand, for many metabolic and nutritional reasons, they are also prone to hyperglycemia. As early as feasible, we start with 2 g/kg/day of proteins and increase the amount by 0.5–1 to 3.5–4 g/kg/day of proteins, which is needed to attain the intrauterine growth rate [55, 56]. It is also important to provide the preterm 25 nonprotein kcal/1 g of proteins. Low blood urea nitrogen (BUN) is a sign of inadequate protein intake, but a high BUN does not correlate well with a high protein intake [57]. A preterm newborn daily loses 1 g of proteins through the kidneys, and a good caloric input with appropriately balanced diet accumulates 2 g of proteins. Thus, improperly balanced nutrition of a newborn can lead to a loss of 15% of protein mass in 2 days [58]. There are eight essential amino acids in parenteral nutrition and six more for the preterm newborn. Adding cysteine to the parenteral nutrition improved nitrogen balance [59], but the addition of glutamine had no clinical impact [60]. Concomitantly with proteins, we administer 20% of intravenous lipids, including essential fatty acids and long-chain n–3 polyunsaturated fatty acids and start with 1 g/kg/day and increase by 0.5 g/kg/day to a maximum of 3–4 g/kg/day [61–63]. Already 0.5 g/kg/day may provide prevention of essential fatty acid deficiency, and the tolerance is guided by triglyceride level of <200 mg/dL. The tolerance is better achieved with the use of continuous infusion of intravenous lipids over 24 h rather than intermittent dosing [64].

To maintain bone health, the newborns need 1.5–2 mmol/kg/day of calcium and the same amount of phosphorus, and 0.18–0.3 mmol/kg/day of magnesium. The optimal weight ratio of calcium and phosphorus is 1.3–1.7:1. Pediatric vitamin formulations of water- and fat-soluble vitamins and trace elements are in use, but they do not provide enough amounts of vitamin A, D and E so we add them enterally if feasible. Vitamin A affects normal eye and lung development, immunity, and cell differentiation. Supplementation of vitamin A in preterm newborns was associated with reduced risk of oxygen requirement [65]. Selenium supplementation prevented short-term morbidity in preterm newborns [66]. Although carnitine supplementation was not associated with weight gain or apnea reduction [67, 68] there are recommendations to add parenteral carnitine to preterm newborns needing parenteral nutrition for more than 2 weeks [69]. Nutritional status can be evaluated by anthropometry, body composition and biochemistry, clinical assessment and quantity, and quality dietary evaluation. Adverse effects of parenteral nutrition include line infection and sepsis, extravasation of parenteral fluid, cholestasis, and bone disease.

To correct the intrauterine growth restriction and achieve appropriate postnatal weight gain, the enteral feeding is also of great significance [70]. It is important to start enteral feeding as early as feasible; in very low birth weight (VLBW) newborns 10–20 mL/kg/day is started in the first 2–5 days, in low birth weight (LBW) newborns in first days [71]. Colostrum acts as the immune therapy for the newborn's intestine. Feeding newborns with minimal volumes of milk is known as trophic feeding, which has many beneficial effects for further feeding, increased hormone secretion, motility, and decreased permeability of the gastrointestinal tract [72]. After a few days of gastrointestinal priming, feedings are increased by 10–20 mL/kg/day. Human milk in comparison with formula resulted in earlier adequate energy intake [73, 74]. Fast advancement of milk volume has no adverse outcome in comparison with slow advancement [71]. Feeding every two hours was superior to feeding every three hours in regards to the time to reach full enteral feeds and better weight gain [75]. Tube feeding can be bolus or continuous and neither is superior [76]. Feeding intolerance can be determined by emesis, gastric residuals, distended, and tender abdomen with changed bowel sounds and stool output, but most of them have little prognostic value [77–80]. The prokinetic erythromycin has not been shown to be effective [81–83]. When the newborn tolerates 100 mL/kg/day or has been consuming mother's milk for 1 week, formula or mother's milk is fortified. The goal of enteral feeding of the preterm newborn is to gain more than 15 g/kg/day.

9. Pain management

Critically ill newborn is confronted with different, more or less painful procedures every day in the NICU. Not every procedure is painful, but the usual response from the newborn is typical —removal of the affected part of the body and crying. The more severe the pain, the more distressful situation is for the newborn. Brain not yet fully developed may receive too many painful stimulations per day, and the tinny newborn may overreact even if the next stimulus is less or even not painful. Newborn Individualized Developmental Care and Assessment Program (NIDCAP) is a method of ensuring an adequate physical environment, reducing overwhelming sensory stimulations, and increasing sensitive parent caregiving, for proper brain growth and development of preterm newborns. Despite non-convincing evidence that NIDCAP improves long-term neurodevelopmental or short-term medical outcome, there is a need for high-quality researches using different techniques to diminish high environmental stress on the premature infants during their treatment in the NICU [84].

Newborns with RDS experience different kinds of pain depending on their morbidities: skin breaking procedures and tissue injury provoke acute or physiological pain, surgery, localized inflammation, and birth trauma cause established pain and diseases like NEC, meningitis, and scalded skin syndrome give rise to prolonged or chronic pain [85]. It has been estimated that sick newborns experience 12–16 procedures each day which are increasingly painful:

1. Routine procedures (physical examination, diaper changes, nasogastric or orogastric insertion, bladder catheterization) [86];
2. Moderately invasive procedures (endotracheal suction, heel lance, venipuncture, arterial puncture, peripherally inserted central catheter placement); and
3. Severely invasive procedures (central venous line placement, chest tube insertion) [87].

Management of pain in newborns with RDS encompasses prevention with first awareness of causing pain with different painful procedures and reduction of painful management of the newborn. The second line includes objective assessment for the detection of pain in each neonate. Thirdly, controlling the pain includes cooperation with parents to diminish pain experience, delivering proper analgesia before expected painful medical care and combining nonpharmacological interventions and pharmacological therapy [88–90].

An important issue in caring for a newborn with RDS is minimal handling or "do not touch" approach. This also enables us to take in mind the possible pain we are going to cause to the newborn with our intended handling and executed procedures. On the other hand, we have to carefully plan the management not to compromise the well-being of the newborn by not performing vital examinations and investigations. By planning the handling of the newborn in limited number of sessions per day, it is possible to disrupt the newborns less times and perform the examinations, nursing care, and blood withdrawal at the same time. We should use laboratory equipment that enables us to analyze several different chemical substances from one small blood sample to reduce the volume of blood taken from the child and avoid iatrogenic anemia. All sick newborns with RDS need intravenous line for fluid, nutritional, antimicrobial, blood pressure, and pain management so a central venous line as soon as possible and for newborns who need several blood investigations per day an artery line should be placed both with appropriate analgesia. With minimally invasive approach, we can gain many data on the well-being of the newborn by noninvasive monitoring with the use of transcutaneous measuring of the oxygen saturation in peripheral arteries and in different organs by the use of near-infrared spectroscopy (NIRS), partial pressures of oxygen, and carbon dioxide in skin capillaries or bilirubin concentrations [85, 89, 91].

For the assessment of pain, different observational scales designed for special newborn population are in use, which encompass many physiological and behavioral variables. Especially with observation of behavior, there is much subjectivity in the assessment procedure. The available assessment scales have proved usable in acute pain, but there is limited applicability of the assessment scales for assessing prolonged pain, pain in extremely low birth weight (ELBW) newborns and in those receiving paralytic agents [85].

First step on the ladder of pain management constitutes the nonpharmacological measures which include sweet peroral solutions, breastfeeding, sucking, skin-to-skin contact, and swaddling with facilitated tucking and sensorial saturation [92]. Combined use of nonpharmacological measures act synergistically [93–95]. Furthermore, when used with pharmacological measures, the pharmacologic use is lesser in frequency and dosage [88, 96]. Sucrose and glucose used before skin-breaking procedures reduced total crying time, lessened changes of physiological variables, and facial expressions and pain scores of multidimensional pain assessment scales [97, 98]. Currently, it is not entirely clear how sweet solutions suppress the responses to painful stimulation; do they only diminish the response to pain or they really influence the pain perception. With repeated dosing, there is a concern on neurodevelopmental outcome in the preterm newborns [99]. Sucrose alone is used for minor procedures, and combined with other analgesics for moderately painful procedures [97]. In cases when physically possible, breastfeeding or mother's milk is at least as effective as sweet solutions [100]. Further on, engaging different body sensors with sensations, like non-nutritive sucking, swaddling, facilitated tucking, rocking, holding, kangaroo care and sensorial saturation, gives the brain other stimuli and therefore the brain has closed door for pain reception [88, 92].

Topical analgesia with the use of Eutectic Mixture of Local Anesthetics (EMLA) or lidocaine alone are used with effect in venous, arterial, and lumbar punctures and also venous, arterial catheter placement, and circumcision. With reasonable dosing, methemoglobinemia is not a significant problem [101].

Systemic analgesia can be provided by nonopioid, nonsteroidal anti-inflammatory agents, opioid analgesics, and sedatives. Paracetamol (acetaminophen) does not diminish pain perception after assisted vaginal birth, heel lance, or eye examination. Paracetamol may diminish the need for morphine after surgical procedures in newborns [102]. We use nonsteroidal anti-inflammatory agents for closing PDA in preterm newborns, but because of their serious adverse effects, like gastrointestinal bleeding, platelet dysfunction and decreased glomerular filtration rate, we do not use them as analgesics in newborns. The most powerful analgesics are opioids, and morphine is the most frequently used, either intermittently for acute pain with invasive procedures or continuously for established pain during artificial ventilation or after surgery. Morphine reduces acute pain after some invasive procedures: central line, tracheal, and chest tube insertion [103, 104], but not heelstick [105] or tracheal suctioning [106, 107]. The NEOPAIN study showed no difference in mortality rate, severe IVH and PVL between ventilated preterm newborns receiving continuous morphine or placebo. The preterm newborns treated with morphine had less pain, but more hypotension, longer duration of artificial ventilation and longer time to full volume feeds [103]. Morphine is safe and effective for treating established pain after surgery in newborns [108, 109]. In extremely preterm newborns, opioid analgesics should be used cautiously [110, 111].

More rapid analgesia with fewer hemodynamic adverse effects is achieved by fentanyl and shorter-acting derivatives, which is suitable for acute invasive procedures in controlled clinical setting like tracheal tube and central line placement [112, 113]. There was no favorable effect on established pain during artificial ventilation of premature newborns using fentanyl [114]. Furthermore, premature newborns treated with continuous fentanyl had prolonged time of artificial ventilation and of meconium passage. Fentanyl is used for treating established pain after surgery and in newborns with pulmonary hypertension.

Ketamine causes analgesia with sedation and amnesia with no effect on respiration and increasing blood pressure and heart rate [115]. It is used in newborns with hemodynamic instability for acute pain with invasive procedures and for established pain during and after surgery [116]. Among sedatives midazolam which can cause prolonged sedation in sick preterm newborns is not recommended for use in preterm newborns [117].

Painful experiences in early childhood may have unfavorable consequences for neurodevelopment [118, 119]. Although there are some data indicating that prolonged use of analgesics in newborns does not influence long-term neurodevelopmental and behavioral outcome [120–122], more recent studies have shown some adverse long-term effects on growth, neurological, and behavioral outcome [123]. A positive autonomic nervous system's stability to pain in neonates with kangaroo care or skin to skin care can be proved by measuring heart rate variability [124, 125].

http://dx.doi.org/10.5772/63386

10. Blood pressure and perfusion management

Systemic blood pressure is dependent on systemic blood flow with cardiac output and systemic vascular resistance. Hypotension ensues in cases of decreased cardiac output as a result of cardiac dysfunction or hypovolemia with inadequate compensation with vasomotor tone, or, decreased vasomotor tone with inadequate compensatory increase in cardiac output. Hypotension, especially in preterms, is difficult to define unequivocally; population-based normative blood pressure data show the increment of blood pressure with increasing gestational and postnatal age, but normal gestational and postnatal age dependent blood pressure range is not known [126]. The physiological principles of blood pressure define autoregulatory threshold where there is loss of autoregulation of blood flow to vital organs, functional threshold where there is loss of cellular function, and ischemic threshold where there is loss of functional integrity [127]. Blood pressure correlates poorly with systemic and cerebral blood flow; therefore, different measurement approaches combined with clinical assessment of adequate perfusion have been investigated for the purpose of better hemodynamic monitoring. Systemic blood flow can be measured by clinician performed ultrasound of the heart and blood vessels with the pressure wave-form analysis and by magnetic resonance imaging (MRI) [128, 129]. Systemic resistance is evaluated by Laser-Doppler technique and by NIRS [130]. Noninvasively, NIRS gives us information about oxygenation of organs, inferring about oxygen delivery, and oxygen demand of certain tissues. The brain activity can continuously be monitored by concomitant use of NIRS and amplitude integrated electroencephalography (EEG) [131, 132].

The blood flow is regulated by cardiac output, carbon dioxide tension, local neuronal and chemical activity, changes in cerebrospinal fluid hydrogen ion concentration, arterial oxygen content, hemoglobin, and blood glucose [133–135]. Accordingly, systemic blood flow can be improved by inotropes or volume, and systemic resistance can be improved by vasopressors and lusitropes. Treatment of neonatal hypotension improves blood pressure, cardiac output, organ blood flow, lactic acidosis, peripheral perfusion, and urine output. Neonatal hypotension endangers cerebral autoregulation and increases morbidity and mortality in preterm newborns [136, 137].

Low systemic blood pressure frequently occurs in the early stages of RDS. Therefore, blood pressure should frequently be measured, either noninvasively or invasively with intravascular line. For volume expansion, after hypovolemia crystalloid or colloid solutions are used [138, 139]. For decreased cardiac output because of cardiac dysfunction, the initial agent is dopamine, later dobutamine, and epinephrine are added [140, 141]. In newborns with refractory hypotension or high-dose inotropic therapy, glucocorticoid therapy increases blood pressure [142, 143]. Different developmental factors affect hemodynamic response to sympathomimetic amines in newborns [144]. Before deciding on a specific therapy of hypotension, potentially reversible causes have to be taken in mind and corrected if possible (measurement error, blood loss, pneumothorax, sepsis, adrenocortical insufficiency).

There is conflicting evidence on the management of hypotension improving clinically meaningful longer-term outcome measures in VLBW newborns, but there are many confounding factors influencing the outcome of management of preterm newborns and studies are weak to show the impact [145–148].

Besides cardiac output, the oxygen supply to the tissues depends also on the content of oxygen in the arteries, which is in the biggest part a function of concentration of hemoglobin. Target values of hemoglobin or hematocrit differ with regards to the gestational and postnatal age of the newborn, the rate of evolution of anemia, the presence of clinical signs of anemia, and the degree of respiratory support [149]. Targeting to lower concentrations of hemoglobin in ELBW newborns might have no effect on short-term outcomes, but may have a negative impact on the longer-tem neurodevelopmental outcome [150, 151]. Anemia can be avoided or postponed by delayed cord clamping or cord milking and also by applications of erythropoietin. Delayed cord clamping and cord milking in preterm newborns was associated with higher hematocrit, fewer transfusions, less IVH, NEC, and no increased need for phototherapy because of jaundice [152–156]. Also, preterm newborns who were receiving erythropoietin received fewer transfusions and had higher cognitive scores at 18–22 months of corrected age [157, 158].

11. PDA management

Shunting blood from the aorta to the pulmonary artery means decreased blood flow in the systemic circulation and low perfusion of peripheral organs and increased blood flow in the pulmonary circulation with RDS, pulmonary edema, BPD, IVH, NEC, and heart failure. Newborns with PDA have higher mortality rate and increased risk of pulmonary edema, hemorrhage, and BPD. The field of management of the PDA is an area in neonatal practice which has, perhaps, changed the most in the last decades and many questions still remain unanswered. The uses of antenatal steroids, postnatal surfactant, and the gentler modes of ventilation with lower oxygen saturation targets may have lowered the incidence and the impact of clinically significant PDA shunt. In VLBV newborns with RDS, PDA is present in 30% [159, 160]. Current management of the PDA generally includes three approaches. Supportive care for newborns with PDA encompasses providing thermal neutrality, using PEEP, keeping hematocrit between 35 and 40%, fluid restriction of 110–130 ml/kg/day, permissive hypercapnia, low oxygen saturation targets and, in case of diuretic need, thiazide diuretics over loop diuretics. If the newborn has poor perfusion, a large left-to-right shunt and remains artificially ventilated for a longer time a course of cyclooxygenase (COX) inhibitors is administered, favoring ibuprofen over indomethacin, because the latter is reducing blood flow to the brain, gastrointestinal tract, and kidneys [161, 162]. Ibuprofen is efficacious for closing PDA given either intravenously or orally [163]. Newborns, who remain artificially ventilated and have failed to respond to COX inhibitor, are candidates for surgical ligation, which has been associated with adverse long-term outcomes [164].

The prophylactic therapy to reduce the incidence of PDA has not been proved to be of benefit. The prophylactic indomethacin has been shown to have no impact on mortality, neurologic impairment, BPD, or NEC although it was associated with reduction of hemodynamically important PDA and severe IVH [165]. The prophylactic ibuprofen has been linked with adverse effects [166, 167].

http://dx.doi.org/10.5772/63386

12. Postnatal supplemental management of respiratory support

Apnea of prematurity is a developmental consequence of immature respiratory center in premature newborns. Besides mechanical ventilation with oxygen supplementation the management of apnea of prematurity encompasses supportive measures like assuring the temperature stability, proper positioning of the newborn's head and neck and ensuring the nasal patency. Methylxanthines stimulate the respiratory drive by increasing the responsiveness of respiratory center to carbon dioxide and decreasing its hypoxic depression. The medicines also have inotropic effects on respiratory muscles [168]. Caffeine is being preferred over theophylline and other agents [169]. Caffeine therapy has been proved to shorten the duration of mechanical ventilation and supplemental oxygen and also reducing the risk of BPD and PDA ligation [170, 171]. The same effects have been shown for prophylactic use of caffeine in very preterm newborns [172, 173]. There have been some positive neurodevelopmental effects of caffeine therapy proved during follow-up of children treated with caffeine during neonatal period [174–176].

The duration of mechanical ventilation can be shortened and the risk of BPD diminished by the use of postnatal tapering course of low- (<0.2 mg/kg/day) or even very low-dose dexamethasone (0.05 mg/kg/day) [177, 178]. Hydrocortisone has been proved to have the same beneficial effects on earlier extubating of mechanically ventilated preterm newborns [179].

13. Conclusion

For the best outcomes of newborns with RDS, besides optimal pulmonary management, it is of extreme importance to have optimal supportive care (**Table 1**) starting prenatally and aiming at newborns being delivered in highly specialized tertiary centers with timing of birth after completion of a course of prenatal steroids. Body temperature should be maintained between 36.5 and 37.5°C. Preterm newborns should be nursed in incubators with high relative humidity (60–80%) and started on intravenous fluids of 70–80 ml/kg/day, later managed individually, based on weight change and serum electrolyte concentrations. Both parenteral and minimal enteral nutrition should be started as early as possible—from day 1—and quickly increased to 3.5 g/kg/day of proteins and 3 g/kg/day of lipids. Proper infection control starts prenatally with administering antibiotics to women with preterm prelabor rupture of membranes, and before labor to those with risk factors for early-onset sepsis. Furthermore, antibiotics are given to newborns with RDS until early-onset sepsis is ruled out. Adequate treatment of pain may be associated with decreased complications and mortality. Sedatives do not provide pain relief and may mask newborn's response to pain. Additionally, proper management of the PDA and hemodynamic support of the circulation with good systemic perfusion and oxygenation are also of utmost importance for the best outcomes of newborns with RDS.

Prenatal care	All the measures to prevent preterm delivery should be taken (counseling, progesterone, antibiotic, magnesium sulfate, tocolysis) If possible, birth should be delayed to allow effect of antenatal steroid therapy to the mother Timely and safe transport of the expectant mother to specialized tertiary centers Appropriate intrapartum antibiotic prophylaxis
Delivery room stabilization	Delayed cord clamping or cord milking at birth Collecting cord blood for diagnostic purposes (hemogram, hemoculture, blood group, virology) Stabilization of the preterm newborn in a plastic bag under a radiant warmer Drying the newborn's skin, providing warmth, positioning the head and clearing the airway, evaluation of respiration and oxygenation of peripheral organs
Supportive care	Nursing the newborn in incubators with heated and humidified air In cases with risk factors for early-onset sepsis and/or clinical and laboratory signs of sepsis antibiotics should be started Insertion of central lines to enable blood withdrawal for diagnostic purposes and parenteral nutrition Careful fluid and electrolyte therapy Early parenteral nutrition and early trophic feeding Minimal handling with clustered care of examination, blood withdrawal and nursing care at the same time but not to overburden the neonate Regular use of appropriate pain assessment scales and proper analgesia before planned procedures Regular measurement of blood pressure and assessment of peripheral perfusion to decide on possible hemodynamic therapy Targeting hemoglobin or hematocrit values in regards to the gestational and postnatal age, the rate of evolution of anemia, the presence of clinical signs of anemia and the degree of respiratory support needed Consideration on the presence and clinical significance of patent ductus arteriosus to decide on possible therapies Caffeine therapy to minimize the need for and duration of ventilation Consideration on postnatal tapering course of low- or very low-dose dexamethasone or hydrocortisone

Adapted from Sweet et al. [1].

Table 1. Summary of recommendations for non-pulmonary management of newborns with respiratory distress.

Author details

Petja Fister[1*] and Štefan Grosek[2,3]

*Address all correspondence to: petja.fister@kclj.si and petja_fister@yahoo.com

1 Department of Neonatology, University Children's Hospital, University Medical Centre Ljubljana, Ljubljana, Slovenia

2 Department of Pediatric Surgery and Intensive Therapy, Surgical Service, University Medical Centre Ljubljana, Ljubljana, Slovenia

3 Department of Pediatrics, Medical Faculty, University of Ljubljana, Ljubljana, Slovenia

References

[1] Sweet DG, Carnielli V, Greisen G, Hallman M, Ozek E, Plavka R, et al. European consensus guidelines on the management of neonatal respiratory distress syndrome in preterm infants—2013 update. Neonatology. 2013;103(4):353–68. doi: 10.1159/000349928.

[2] Stoll BJ, Hansen NI, Bell EF, Shankaran S, Laptook AR, Walsh MC, et al. Neonatal outcomes of extremely preterm infants from the NICHD Neonatal Research Network. Pediatrics. 2010;126(3):443–56. doi:10.1542/peds.2009–2959.

[3] Costeloe KL, Hennessy EM, Haider S, Stacey F, Marlow N, Draper ES. Short term outcomes after extreme preterm birth in England: comparison of two birth cohorts in 1995 and 2006 (the EPICure studies). BMJ. 2012;345:e7976. doi:10.1136/bmj.e7976.

[4] Robbins CL, Zapata LB, Farr SL, Kroelinger CD, Morrow B, Ahluwalia I, et al. Core state preconception health indicators—pregnancy risk assessment monitoring system and behavioral risk factor surveillance system, 2009. MMWR Surveill Summ. 2014;63(3):1–62.

[5] Di Renzo GC, Roura LC, Facchinetti F, Antsaklis A, Breborowicz G, Gratacos E, et al. Guidelines for the management of spontaneous preterm labor: identification of spontaneous preterm labor, diagnosis of preterm premature rupture of membranes, and preventive tools for preterm birth. J Matern Fetal Neonatal Med. 2011;24(5):659–67. doi:10.3109/14767058.2011.553694.

[6] Rautava L, Eskelinen J, Häkkinen U, Lehtonen L, Group PPIS. 5-year morbidity among very preterm infants in relation to level of hospital care. JAMA Pediatr. 2013;167(1):40–6. doi:10.1001/jamapediatrics.2013.415.

[7] Kenyon S, Boulvain M, Neilson J. Antibiotics for preterm rupture of membranes. Cochrane Database Syst Rev. 2010(8):CD001058. doi:10.1002/14651858.CD001058.pub2.

[8] Hutzal C, Boyle E, Kenyon S, Nash J, Winsor S, Taylor D, et al. Use of antibiotics for the treatment of preterm parturition and prevention of neonatal morbidity: a metaanalysis. Am J Obstet Gynecol. 2008;199(6):620.e1–8. doi:10.1016/j.ajog.2008.07.008.

[9] ACOG Committee Opinion No. 445: antibiotics for preterm labor. Obstet Gynecol. 2009;114(5):1159–60. doi:10.1097/AOG.0b013e3181c33c86.

[10] Doyle L, Crowther C, Middleton P, Marret S, Rouse D. Magnesium sulphate for women at risk of preterm birth for neuroprotection of the fetus. Cochrane Database Syst Rev. 2009;(1):CD004661. doi:10.1002/14651858.CD004661.pub3.

[11] Haas DM, Caldwell DM, Kirkpatrick P, McIntosh JJ, Welton NJ. Tocolytic therapy for preterm delivery: systematic review and network meta-analysis. BMJ. 2012;345:e6226. doi:10.1136/bmj.e6226.

[12] Roberts D, Dalziel S. Antenatal corticosteroids for accelerating fetal lung maturation for women at risk of preterm birth. Cochrane Database Syst Rev. 2006;(3):CD004454.

[13] Sotiriadis A, Makrydimas G, Papatheodorou S, Ioannidis J. Corticosteroids for preventing neonatal respiratory morbidity after elective caesarean section at term. Cochrane Database Syst Rev. 2009;(4):CD006614. doi: 10.1002/14651858.CD006614.pub2.

[14] Crowther C, McKinlay C, Middleton P, Harding J. Repeat doses of prenatal corticosteroids for women at risk of preterm birth for improving neonatal health outcomes. Cochrane Database Syst Rev. 2011;(6):CD003935. doi: 10.1002/14651858.CD003935.pub3.

[15] Thomas W, Speer CP. Chorioamnionitis: important risk factor or innocent bystander for neonatal outcome? Neonatology. 2011;99(3):177–87. doi:10.1159/000320170.

[16] Girard S, Kadhim H, Roy M, Lavoie K, Brochu M, Larouche A, et al. Role of perinatal inflammation in cerebral palsy. Pediatr Neurol. 2009;40(3):168–74. doi:10.1016/j.pediatrneurol.2008.09.016.

[17] Baker CJ, Byington CL, Polin RA, Diseases CoI, Newborn CoFa. Policy statement—recommendations for the prevention of perinatal group B streptococcal (GBS) disease. Pediatrics. 2011;128(3):611–6. doi:10.1542/peds.2011-1466.

[18] Grosek S, Mlakar G, Vidmar I, Ihan A, Primozic J. Heart rate and leukocytes after air and ground transportation in artificially ventilated neonates: a prospective observational study. Intensive Care Med. 2009;35(1):161–5. doi:10.1007/s00134-008-1256-8.

[19] de Almeida M, Guinsburg R, Sancho G, Rosa I, Lamy Z, Martinez F, et al. Hypothermia and early neonatal mortality in preterm infants. J Pediatr. 2014;164(2):271–5.e1. doi: 10.1016/j.jpeds.2013.09.049.

[20] Miller SS, Lee HC, Gould JB. Hypothermia in very low birth weight infants: distribution, risk factors and outcomes. J Perinatol. 2011;31(Suppl 1):S49–56. doi:10.1038/jp.2010.177.

[21] Laptook AR, Salhab W, Bhaskar B, Network NR. Admission temperature of low birth weight infants: predictors and associated morbidities. Pediatrics. 2007;119(3):e643–9.

[22] McCall E, Alderdice F, Halliday H, Jenkins J, Vohra S. Interventions to prevent hypothermia at birth in preterm and/or low birthweight infants. Cochrane Database Syst Rev. 2010;(3):CD004210. doi:10.1002/14651858.CD004210.pub4.

[23] Reilly MC, Vohra S, Rac VE, Dunn M, Ferrelli K, Kiss A, et al. Randomized trial of occlusive wrap for heat loss prevention in preterm infants. J Pediatr. 2015;166(2):262–8.e2. doi:10.1016/j.jpeds.2014.09.068.

[24] Doglioni N, Cavallin F, Mardegan V, Palatron S, Filippone M, Vecchiato L, et al. Total body polyethylene wraps for preventing hypothermia in preterm infants: a randomized trial. J Pediatr. 2014;165(2):261–6.e1. doi:10.1016/j.jpeds.2014.04.010.

[25] Leadford AE, Warren JB, Manasyan A, Chomba E, Salas AA, Schelonka R, et al. Plastic bags for prevention of hypothermia in preterm and low birth weight infants. Pediatrics. 2013;132(1):e128–34. doi:10.1542/peds.2012-2030.

[26] Trevisanuto D, Doglioni N, Cavallin F, Parotto M, Micaglio M, Zanardo V. Heat loss prevention in very preterm infants in delivery rooms: a prospective, randomized, controlled trial of polyethylene caps. J Pediatr. 2010;156(6):914–7, 7.e1. doi:10.1016/j.jpeds.2009.12.021.

[27] Cramer K, Wiebe N, Hartling L, Crumley E, Vohra S. Heat loss prevention: a systematic review of occlusive skin wrap for premature neonates. J Perinatol. 2005;25(12):763–9.

[28] Deguines C, Décima P, Pelletier A, Dégrugilliers L, Ghyselen L, Tourneux P. Variations in incubator temperature and humidity management: a survey of current practice. Acta Paediatr. 2012;101(3):230–5. doi:10.1111/j.1651-2227.2011.02492.x.

[29] Jia Y, Lin Z, Lv H, Li Y, Green R, Lin J. Effect of delivery room temperature on the admission temperature of premature infants: a randomized controlled trial. J Perinatol. 2013;33(4):264–7. doi:10.1038/jp.2012.100.

[30] Russo A, McCready M, Torres L, Theuriere C, Venturini S, Spaight M, et al. Reducing hypothermia in preterm infants following delivery. Pediatrics. 2014;133(4):E1055–E62. doi:10.1542/peds.2013-2544.

[31] Moore E, Anderson G, Bergman N, Dowswell T. Early skin-to-skin contact for mothers and their healthy newborn infants. Cochrane Database Syst Rev. 2012;(5):CD003519. doi:10.1002/14651858.CD003519.pub3.

[32] Karlsson V, Heinemann A, Sjors G, Nykvist K, Agren J. Early skin-to-skin care in extremely preterm infants: thermal balance and care environment. J Pediatr. 2012;161(3):422–6. doi:10.1016/j.jpeds.2012.02.034.

[33] Meyer M, Hou D, Ishrar N, Ishrar N, te Pas A. Initial respiratory support with cold, dry gas versus heated humidified gas and admission temperature of preterm infants. J Pediatr. 2015;166(2):245–50.e1. doi:10.1016/j.jpeds.2014.09.049.

[34] Pas A, Lopriore E, Dito I, Morley C, Walther F. Humidified and heated air during stabilization at birth improves temperature in preterm infants. Pediatrics. 2010;125(6):E1427–E32. doi:10.1542/peds.2009-2656.

[35] Stoll B, Hansen N, Sanchez P, Faix R, Poindexter B, Van Meurs K, et al. Early onset neonatal sepsis: the burden of Group B *Streptococcal* and *E. coli* disease continues. Pediatrics. 2011;127(5):817–26. doi:10.1542/peds.2010-2217.

[36] Ohlsson A, Shah V. Intrapartum antibiotics for known maternal Group B streptococcal colonization. Cochrane Database Syst Rev. 2014;(6):CD007467. doi: 10.1002/14651858.CD007467.pub4.

[37] Tzialla C, Borghesi A, Perotti GF, Garofoli F, Manzoni P, Stronati M. Use and misuse of antibiotics in the neonatal intensive care unit. J Matern Fetal Neonatal Med. 2012;25(Suppl 4):35–7. doi:10.3109/14767058.2012.714987.

[38] Kuppala V, Meinzen-Derr J, Morrow A, Schibler K. Prolonged initial empirical antibiotic treatment is associated with adverse outcomes in premature infants. J Pediatr. 2011;159(5):720–5. doi:10.1016/j.jpeds.2011.05.033.

[39] Auriti C, Ravà L, Di Ciommo V, Ronchetti MP, Orzalesi M. Short antibiotic prophylaxis for bacterial infections in a neonatal intensive care unit: a randomized controlled trial. J Hosp Infect. 2005;59(4):292–8.

[40] Stoll BJ, Hansen N, Fanaroff AA, Wright LL, Carlo WA, Ehrenkranz RA, et al. Late-onset sepsis in very low birth weight neonates: the experience of the NICHD Neonatal Research Network. Pediatrics. 2002;110(2 Pt 1):285–91.

[41] Stoll BJ, Hansen NI, Adams-Chapman I, Fanaroff AA, Hintz SR, Vohr B, et al. Neurodevelopmental and growth impairment among extremely low-birth-weight infants with neonatal infection. JAMA. 2004;292(19):2357–65.

[42] Roberts KB. Fluid and electrolytes: parenteral fluid therapy. Pediatr Rev. 2001;22(11): 380–7.

[43] Baumgart S, Costarino AT. Water and electrolyte metabolism of the micropremie. Clin Perinatol. 2000;27(1):131–46, vi–vii.

[44] Omar SA, DeCristofaro JD, Agarwal BI, La Gamma EF. Effects of prenatal steroids on water and sodium homeostasis in extremely low birth weight neonates. Pediatrics. 1999;104(3 Pt 1):482–8.

[45] Omar SA, DeCristofaro JD, Agarwal BI, LaGamma EF. Effect of prenatal steroids on potassium balance in extremely low birth weight neonates. Pediatrics. 2000;106(3):561–7.

[46] Bell EF, Acarregui MJ. Restricted versus liberal water intake for preventing morbidity and mortality in preterm infants. Cochrane Database Syst Rev. 2014;12:CD000503. doi: 10.1002/14651858.CD000503.pub3.

[47] Stewart A, Brion LP, Soll R. Diuretics for respiratory distress syndrome in preterm infants. Cochrane Database Syst Rev. 2011;(12):CD001454. doi: 10.1002/14651858.CD001454.pub3.

[48] Canani RB, Costanzo MD, Leone L, Bedogni G, Brambilla P, Cianfarani S, et al. Epigenetic mechanisms elicited by nutrition in early life. Nutr Res Rev. 2011;24(2):198–205. doi:10.1017/S0954422411000102.

[49] Stephens BE, Walden RV, Gargus RA, Tucker R, McKinley L, Mance M, et al. First-week protein and energy intakes are associated with 18-month developmental outcomes in extremely low birth weight infants. Pediatrics. 2009;123(5):1337–43. doi:10.1542/peds.2008-0211.

[50] Christmann V, Visser R, Engelkes M, de Grauw AM, van Goudoever JB, van Heijst AF. The enigma to achieve normal postnatal growth in preterm infants—using parenteral or enteral nutrition? Acta Paediatr. 2013;102(5):471–9. doi:10.1111/apa.12188.

[51] Moyses HE, Johnson MJ, Leaf AA, Cornelius VR. Early parenteral nutrition and growth outcomes in preterm infants: a systematic review and meta-analysis. Am J Clin Nutr. 2013;97(4):816–26. doi:10.3945/ajcn.112.042028.

[52] Hay WW. Aggressive nutrition of the preterm infant. Curr Pediatr Rep. 2013;1(4): 229-39. doi:10.1007/s40124-013-0026-4.

[53] Parish A, Bhatia J. Early aggressive nutrition for the premature infant. Neonatology. 2008;94(3):211–4. doi:10.1159/000143724.

[54] Ehrenkranz RA. Early, aggressive nutritional management for very low birth weight infants: what is the evidence? Semin Perinatol. 2007;31(2):48–55.

[55] Trivedi A, Sinn JK. Early versus late administration of amino acids in preterm infants receiving parenteral nutrition. Cochrane Database Syst Rev. 2013;7:CD008771. doi: 10.1002/14651858.CD008771.pub2.

[56] Klein CJ. Nutrient requirements for preterm infant formulas. J Nutr. 2002;132(6 Suppl 1):1395S–577S.

[57] Burattini I, Bellagamba MP, Spagnoli C, D'Ascenzo R, Mazzoni N, Peretti A, et al. Targeting 2.5 versus 4 g/kg/day of amino acids for extremely low birth weight infants: a randomized clinical trial. J Pediatr. 2013;163(5):1278–82.e1. doi:10.1016/j.jpeds.2013.06.075.

[58] Porcelli PJ, Jr., Sisk PM. Increased parenteral amino acid administration to extremely low-birth-weight infants during early postnatal life. J Pediatr Gastroenterol Nutr. 2002;34(2):174–9.

[59] Soghier LM, Brion LP. Cysteine, cystine or N-acetylcysteine supplementation in parenterally fed neonates. Cochrane Database Syst Rev. 2006;(4):CD004869.

[60] Tubman TR, Thompson SW, McGuire W. Glutamine supplementation to prevent morbidity and mortality in preterm infants. Cochrane Database Syst Rev. 2008;(1):CD001457. doi:10.1002/14651858.CD001457.pub3.

[61] Vlaardingerbroek H, Vermeulen MJ, Rook D, van den Akker CH, Dorst K, Wattimena JL, et al. Safety and efficacy of early parenteral lipid and high-dose amino acid administration to very low birth weight infants. J Pediatr. 2013;163(3):638–44.e1–5. doi:10.1016/j.jpeds.2013.03.059.

[62] Simmer K, Rao SC. Early introduction of lipids to parenterally-fed preterm infants. Cochrane Database Syst Rev. 2005;(2):CD005256.

[63] Simmer K, Patole SK, Rao SC. Long-chain polyunsaturated fatty acid supplementation in infants born at term. Cochrane Database Syst Rev. 2011;(12):CD000376. doi:10.1002/14651858.CD000376.pub3.

[64] Drenckpohl D, McConnell C, Gaffney S, Niehaus M, Macwan KS. Randomized trial of very low birth weight infants receiving higher rates of infusion of intravenous fat emulsions during the first week of life. Pediatrics. 2008;122(4):743–51. doi:10.1542/peds.2007-2282.

[65] Darlow BA, Graham PJ. Vitamin A supplementation to prevent mortality and short- and long-term morbidity in very low birthweight infants. Cochrane Database Syst Rev. 2011;(10):CD000501. doi:10.1002/14651858.CD000501.pub3.

[66] Darlow BA, Austin NC. Selenium supplementation to prevent short-term morbidity in preterm neonates. Cochrane Database Syst Rev. 2003;(4):CD003312.

[67] Pande S, Brion LP, Campbell DE, Gayle Y, Esteban-Cruciani NV. Lack of effect of L-carnitine supplementation on weight gain in very preterm infants. J Perinatol. 2005;25(7):470–7.

[68] Kumar M, Kabra NS, Paes B. Carnitine supplementation for preterm infants with recurrent apnea. Cochrane Database Syst Rev. 2004;(4):CD004497.

[69] Martin CR, Brown YF, Ehrenkranz RA, O'Shea TM, Allred EN, Belfort MB, et al. Nutritional practices and growth velocity in the first month of life in extremely premature infants. Pediatrics. 2009;124(2):649–57. doi:10.1542/peds.2008-3258.

[70] Agostoni C, Buonocore G, Carnielli VP, De Curtis M, Darmaun D, Decsi T, et al. Enteral nutrient supply for preterm infants: commentary from the European Society of Paediatric Gastroenterology, Hepatology and Nutrition Committee on Nutrition. J Pediatr Gastroenterol Nutr. 2010;50(1):85–91. doi:10.1097/MPG.0b013e3181adaee0.

[71] Morgan J, Young L, McGuire W. Slow advancement of enteral feed volumes to prevent necrotising enterocolitis in very low birth weight infants. Cochrane Database Syst Rev. 2015;10:CD001241. doi:10.1002/14651858.CD001241.pub6.

[72] Morgan J, Bombell S, McGuire W. Early trophic feeding versus enteral fasting for very preterm or very low birth weight infants. Cochrane Database Syst Rev. 2013;3:CD000504. doi:10.1002/14651858.CD000504.pub4.

[73] Basuki F, Hadiati DR, Turner T, McDonald S, Hakimi M. Dilute versus full strength formula in exclusively formula-fed preterm or low birth weight infants. Cochrane Database Syst Rev. 2013;11:CD007263. doi:10.1002/14651858.CD007263.pub2.

[74] Sisk PM, Lovelady CA, Gruber KJ, Dillard RG, O'Shea TM. Human milk consumption and full enteral feeding among infants who weigh ≤1250 grams. Pediatrics. 2008;121(6):e1528–33. doi:10.1542/peds.2007-2110.

[75] DeMauro SB, Abbasi S, Lorch S. The impact of feeding interval on feeding outcomes in very low birth-weight infants. J Perinatol. 2011;31(7):481–6. doi:10.1038/jp.2010.153.

[76] Premji SS, Chessell L. Continuous nasogastric milk feeding versus intermittent bolus milk feeding for premature infants less than 1500 grams. Cochrane Database Syst Rev. 2011(11):CD001819. doi:10.1002/14651858.CD001819.pub2.

[77] Jadcherla SR, Kliegman RM. Studies of feeding intolerance in very low birth weight infants: definition and significance. Pediatrics. 2002;109(3):516–7.

[78] Mihatsch WA, von Schoenaich P, Fahnenstich H, Dehne N, Ebbecke H, Plath C, et al. The significance of gastric residuals in the early enteral feeding advancement of extremely low birth weight infants. Pediatrics. 2002;109(3):457–9.

[79] Mihatsch WA, Högel J, Pohlandt F. Hydrolysed protein accelerates the gastrointestinal transport of formula in preterm infants. Acta Paediatr. 2001;90(2):196–8.

[80] Moody GJ, Schanler RJ, Lau C, Shulman RJ. Feeding tolerance in premature infants fed fortified human milk. J Pediatr Gastroenterol Nutr. 2000;30(4):408–12.

[81] Aly H, Abdel-Hady H, Khashaba M, El-Badry N. Erythromycin and feeding intolerance in premature infants: a randomized trial. J Perinatol. 2007;27(1):39–43.

[82] Nuntnarumit P, Kiatchoosakun P, Tantiprapa W, Boonkasidecha S. Efficacy of oral erythromycin for treatment of feeding intolerance in preterm infants. J Pediatr. 2006;148(5):600–5.

[83] Patole S, Rao S, Doherty D. Erythromycin as a prokinetic agent in preterm neonates: a systematic review. Arch Dis Child Fetal Neonatal Ed. 2005;90(4):F301–6.

[84] Ohlsson A, Jacobs SE. NIDCAP: a systematic review and meta-analyses of randomized controlled trials. Pediatrics. 2013;131(3):e881–93. doi:10.1542/peds.2012-2121.

[85] Committee On Fetus And Newborn And Section On Anesthesiology And Pain Medicine. Prevention and management of procedural pain in the neonate: an update. Pediatrics. 2016;137(2):1–13. doi:10.1542/peds.2015-4271.

[86] Pereira-Da-Silva L, Bergmans KI, van Kerkhoven LA, Leal F, Virella D, Videira-Amaral JM. Reducing discomfort while measuring crown-heel length in neonates. Acta Paediatr. 2006;95(6):742–6.

[87] Anand KJ, Aranda JV, Berde CB, Buckman S, Capparelli EV, Carlo W, et al. Summary proceedings from the neonatal pain-control group. Pediatrics. 2006;117(3 Pt 2):S9–S22.

[88] Bellieni CV, Buonocore G. Neonatal pain treatment: ethical to be effective. J Perinatol. 2008;28(2):87–8. doi:10.1038/sj.jp.7211899.

[89] Sharek PJ, Powers R, Koehn A, Anand KJ. Evaluation and development of potentially better practices to improve pain management of neonates. Pediatrics. 2006;118(Suppl 2):S78–86.

[90] Lago P, Garetti E, Merazzi D, Pieragostini L, Ancora G, Pirelli A, et al. Guidelines for procedural pain in the newborn. Acta Paediatr. 2009;98(6):932–9.

[91] Aranda JV, Carlo W, Hummel P, Thomas R, Lehr VT, Anand KJ. Analgesia and sedation during mechanical ventilation in neonates. Clin Ther. 2005;27(6):877–99.

[92] Pillai Riddell RR, Racine NM, Gennis HG, Turcotte K, Uman LS, Horton RE, et al. Non-pharmacological management of infant and young child procedural pain. Cochrane Database Syst Rev. 2015;12:CD006275. doi:10.1002/14651858.CD006275.pub3.

[93] Marín Gabriel M, del Rey Hurtado de Mendoza B, Jiménez Figueroa L, Medina V, Iglesias Fernández B, Vázquez Rodríguez M, et al. Analgesia with breastfeeding in addition to skin-to-skin contact during heel prick. Arch Dis Child Fetal Neonatal Ed. 2013;98(6):F499–503. doi:10.1136/archdischild-2012-302921.

[94] Cignacco EL, Sellam G, Stoffel L, Gerull R, Nelle M, Anand KJ, et al. Oral sucrose and "facilitated tucking" for repeated pain relief in preterms: a randomized controlled trial. Pediatrics. 2012;129(2):299–308. doi:10.1542/peds.2011-1879.

[95] Chermont AG, Falcão LF, de Souza Silva EH, de Cássia Xavier Balda R, Guinsburg R. Skin-to-skin contact and/or oral 25% dextrose for procedural pain relief for term newborn infants. Pediatrics. 2009;124(6):e1101–7. doi:10.1542/peds.2009-0993.

[96] Golianu B, Krane E, Seybold J, Almgren C, Anand KJ. Non-pharmacological techniques for pain management in neonates. Semin Perinatol. 2007;31(5):318–22.

[97] Stevens B, Yamada J, Lee GY, Ohlsson A. Sucrose for analgesia in newborn infants undergoing painful procedures. Cochrane Database Syst Rev. 2013;1:CD001069. doi: 10.1002/14651858.CD001069.pub4.

[98] Okan F, Coban A, Ince Z, Yapici Z, Can G. Analgesia in preterm newborns: the comparative effects of sucrose and glucose. Eur J Pediatr. 2007;166(10):1017–24.

[99] Johnston CC, Filion F, Snider L, Majnemer A, Limperopoulos C, Walker CD, et al. Routine sucrose analgesia during the first week of life in neonates younger than 31 weeks' postconceptional age. Pediatrics. 2002;110(3):523–8.

[100] Shah PS, Herbozo C, Aliwalas LL, Shah VS. Breastfeeding or breast milk for procedural pain in neonates. Cochrane Database Syst Rev. 2012;12:CD004950. doi: 10.1002/14651858.CD004950.pub3.

[101] Taddio A, Ohlsson A, Ohlsson K. WITHDRAWN: Lidocaine–prilocaine cream for analgesia during circumcision in newborn boys. Cochrane Database Syst Rev. 2015;4:CD000496. doi:10.1002/14651858.CD000496.pub2.

[102] Ohlsson A, Shah P. Paracetamol (acetaminophen) for prevention or treatment of pain in newborns. Cochrane Database Syst Rev. 2015;(6):CD011219. doi: 10.1002/14651858.CD011219.pub2.

[103] Anand KJ, Hall RW, Desai N, Shephard B, Bergqvist LL, Young TE, et al. Effects of morphine analgesia in ventilated preterm neonates: primary outcomes from the NEOPAIN randomised trial. Lancet. 2004;363(9422):1673–82.

[104] Taddio A, Lee C, Yip A, Parvez B, McNamara PJ, Shah V. Intravenous morphine and topical tetracaine for treatment of pain in [corrected] neonates undergoing central line placement. JAMA. 2006;295(7):793–800.

[105] Carbajal R, Lenclen R, Jugie M, Paupe A, Barton BA, Anand KJ. Morphine does not provide adequate analgesia for acute procedural pain among preterm neonates. Pediatrics. 2005;115(6):1494–500.

[106] Anand KJ, Anderson BJ, Holford NH, Hall RW, Young T, Shephard B, et al. Morphine pharmacokinetics and pharmacodynamics in preterm and term neonates: secondary results from the NEOPAIN trial. Br J Anaesth. 2008;101(5):680–9. doi:10.1093/bja/aen248.

[107] Simons SH, van Dijk M, van Lingen RA, Roofthooft D, Duivenvoorden HJ, Jongeneel N, et al. Routine morphine infusion in preterm newborns who received ventilatory support: a randomized controlled trial. JAMA. 2003;290(18):2419–27.

[108] El Sayed MF, Taddio A, Fallah S, De Silva N, Moore AM. Safety profile of morphine following surgery in neonates. J Perinatol. 2007;27(7):444–7.

[109] Rouss K, Gerber A, Albisetti M, Hug M, Bernet V. Long-term subcutaneous morphine administration after surgery in newborns. J Perinat Med. 2007;35(1):79–81.

[110] Hall RW, Boyle E, Young T. Do ventilated neonates require pain management? Semin Perinatol. 2007;31(5):289–97.

[111] Hall RW, Kronsberg SS, Barton BA, Kaiser JR, Anand KJ, Group NTI. Morphine, hypotension, and adverse outcomes among preterm neonates: who's to blame? Secondary results from the NEOPAIN trial. Pediatrics. 2005;115(5):1351–9.

[112] Pereira e Silva Y, Gomez RS, Marcatto JeO, Maximo TA, Barbosa RF, Simões e Silva AC. Morphine versus remifentanil for intubating preterm neonates. Arch Dis Child Fetal Neonatal Ed. 2007;92(4):F293–4.

[113] Roberts KD, Leone TA, Edwards WH, Rich WD, Finer NN. Premedication for nonemergent neonatal intubations: a randomized, controlled trial comparing atropine and fentanyl to atropine, fentanyl, and mivacurium. Pediatrics. 2006;118(4):1583–91.

[114] Ancora G, Lago P, Garetti E, Pirelli A, Merazzi D, Mastrocola M, et al. Efficacy and safety of continuous infusion of fentanyl for pain control in preterm newborns on mechanical ventilation. J Pediatr. 2013;163(3):645–51.e1. doi:10.1016/j.jpeds.2013.02.039.

[115] Hall RW, Shbarou RM. Drugs of choice for sedation and analgesia in the neonatal ICU. Clin Perinatol. 2009;36(2):215–26, vii. doi:10.1016/j.clp.2009.04.001.

[116] Saarenmaa E, Neuvonen PJ, Huttunen P, Fellman V. Ketamine for procedural pain relief in newborn infants. Arch Dis Child Fetal Neonatal Ed. 2001;85(1):F53–6.

[117] Ng E, Taddio A, Ohlsson A. Intravenous midazolam infusion for sedation of infants in the neonatal intensive care unit. Cochrane Database Syst Rev. 2012;6:CD002052. doi:10.1002/14651858.CD002052.pub2.

[118] Ranger M, Chau CM, Garg A, Woodward TS, Beg MF, Bjornson B, et al. Neonatal pain-related stress predicts cortical thickness at age 7 years in children born very preterm. PLoS One. 2013;8(10):e76702. doi:10.1371/journal.pone.0076702.

[119] Anand KJ, Palmer FB, Papanicolaou AC. Repetitive neonatal pain and neurocognitive abilities in ex-preterm children. Pain. 2013;154(10):1899–901. doi:10.1016/j.pain.2013.06.027.

[120] de Graaf J, van Lingen RA, Simons SH, Anand KJ, Duivenvoorden HJ, Weisglas-Kuperus N, et al. Long-term effects of routine morphine infusion in mechanically ventilated neonates on children's functioning: five-year follow-up of a randomized controlled trial. Pain. 2011;152(6):1391–7. doi:10.1016/j.pain.2011.02.017.

[121] Bellù R, de Waal K, Zanini R. Opioids for neonates receiving mechanical ventilation: a systematic review and meta-analysis. Arch Dis Child Fetal Neonatal Ed. 2010;95(4):F241–51. doi:10.1136/adc.2008.150318.

[122] Rozé JC, Denizot S, Carbajal R, Ancel PY, Kaminski M, Arnaud C, et al. Prolonged sedation and/or analgesia and 5-year neurodevelopment outcome in very preterm infants: results from the EPIPAGE cohort. Arch Pediatr Adolesc Med. 2008;162(8):728–33. doi:10.1001/archpedi.162.8.728.

[123] Ferguson SA, Ward WL, Paule MG, Hall RW, Anand KJ. A pilot study of preemptive morphine analgesia in preterm neonates: effects on head circumference, social behavior, and response latencies in early childhood. Neurotoxicol Teratol. 2012;34(1):47–55. doi:10.1016/j.ntt.2011.10.008.

[124] Cong X, Cusson RM, Walsh S, Hussain N, Ludington-Hoe SM, Zhang D. Effects of skin-to-skin contact on autonomic pain responses in preterm infants. J Pain. 2012;13(7):636–45. doi:10.1016/j.jpain.2012.02.008.

[125] Cong X, Ludington-Hoe SM, McCain G, Fu P. Kangaroo Care modifies preterm infant heart rate variability in response to heel stick pain: pilot study. Early Hum Dev. 2009;85(9):561–7. doi:10.1016/j.earlhumdev.2009.05.012.

[126] Batton B, Li L, Newman NS, Das A, Watterberg KL, Yoder BA, et al. Evolving blood pressure dynamics for extremely preterm infants. J Perinatol. 2014;34(4):301–5. doi: 10.1038/jp.2014.6.

[127] Rhee CJ, Fraser CD, Kibler K, Easley RB, Andropoulos DB, Czosnyka M, et al. The ontogeny of cerebrovascular pressure autoregulation in premature infants. J Perinatol. 2014;34(12):926–31. doi:10.1038/jp.2014.122.

[128] Kluckow M, Evans N. Superior vena cava flow in newborn infants: a novel marker of systemic blood flow. Arch Dis Child Fetal Neonatal Ed. 2000;82(3):F182–7.

[129] Evans N, Kluckow M, Simmons M, Osborn D. Which to measure, systemic or organ blood flow? Middle cerebral artery and superior vena cava flow in very preterm infants. Arch Dis Child Fetal Neonatal Ed. 2002;87(3):F181–4.

[130] Soleymani S, Borzage M, Seri I. Hemodynamic monitoring in neonates: advances and challenges. J Perinatol. 2010;30(Suppl):S38–45. doi:10.1038/jp.2010.101.

[131] Tataranno ML, Alderliesten T, de Vries LS, Groenendaal F, Toet MC, Lemmers PM, et al. Early oxygen-utilization and brain activity in preterm infants. PLoS One. 2015;10(5):e0124623. Doi:10.1371/journal.pone.0124623.

[132] Pichler G, Avian A, Binder C, Zotter H, Schmölzer GM, Morris N, et al. aEEG and NIRS during transition and resuscitation after birth: promising additional tools; an observational study. Resuscitation. 2013;84(7):974–8. Doi:10.1016/j.resuscitation.2012.12.025.

[133] Kaiser JR, Gauss CH, Williams DK. The effects of hypercapnia on cerebral autoregulation in ventilated very low birth weight infants. Pediatr Res. 2005;58(5):931–5.

[134] Pellicer A, Valverde E, Elorza MD, Madero R, Gayá F, Quero J, et al. Cardiovascular support for low birth weight infants and cerebral hemodynamics: a randomized, blinded, clinical trial. Pediatrics. 2005;115(6):1501–12.

[135] Kusaka T, Okubo K, Nagano K, Isobe K, Itoh S. Cerebral distribution of cardiac output in newborn infants. Arch Dis Child Fetal Neonatal Ed. 2005;90(1):F77–8.

[136] Faust K, Härtel C, PreuيM, Rabe H, Roll C, Emeis M, et al. Short-term outcome of very-low-birthweight infants with arterial hypotension in the first 24 h of life. Arch Dis Child Fetal Neonatal Ed. 2015;100(5):F388–92. Doi:10.1136/archdischild-2014-306483.

[137] Munro MJ, Walker AM, Barfield CP. Hypotensive extremely low birth weight infants have reduced cerebral blood flow. Pediatrics. 2004;114(6):1591–6.

[138] Lynch SK, Mullett MD, Graeber JE, Polak MJ. A comparison of albumin-bolus therapy versus normal saline-bolus therapy for hypotension in neonates. J Perinatol. 2008;28(1): 29–33.

[139] Osborn DA, Evans N. Early volume expansion for prevention of morbidity and mortality in very preterm infants. Cochrane Database Syst Rev. 2004;(2):CD002055.

[140] Subhedar NV, Shaw NJ. Dopamine versus dobutamine for hypotensive preterm infants. Cochrane Database Syst Rev. 2003;(3):CD001242.

[141] Sassano-Higgins S, Friedlich P, Seri I. A meta-analysis of dopamine use in hypotensive preterm infants: blood pressure and cerebral hemodynamics. J Perinatol. 2011;31(10): 647–55. Doi:10.1038/jp.2011.2.

[142] Ibrahim H, Sinha IP, Subhedar NV. Corticosteroids for treating hypotension in preterm infants. Cochrane Database Syst Rev. 2011;(12):CD003662. Doi: 10.1002/14651858.CD003662.pub4.

[143] Finer NN, Powers RJ, Ou CH, Durand D, Wirtschafter D, Gould JB, et al. Prospective evaluation of postnatal steroid administration: a 1-year experience from the California Perinatal Quality Care Collaborative. Pediatrics. 2006;117(3):704–13.

[144] Noori S, Seri I. Neonatal blood pressure support: the use of inotropes, lusitropes, and other vasopressor agents. Clin Perinatol. 2012;39(1):221–38. Doi:10.1016/j.clp. 2011.12.010.

[145] Alderliesten T, Lemmers PM, van Haastert IC, de Vries LS, Bonestroo HJ, Baerts W, et al. Hypotension in preterm neonates: low blood pressure alone does not affect neurodevelopmental outcome. J Pediatr. 2014;164(5):986–91. Doi:10.1016/j.jpeds.2013.12.042.

[146] Batton B, Li L, Newman NS, Das A, Watterberg KL, Yoder BA, et al. Use of antihypotensive therapies in extremely preterm infants. Pediatrics. 2013;131(6):e1865–73. Doi: 10.1542/peds.2012-2779.

[147] Batton B, Zhu X, Fanaroff J, Kirchner HL, Berlin S, Wilson-Costello D, et al. Blood pressure, anti-hypotensive therapy, and neurodevelopment in extremely preterm infants. J Pediatr. 2009;154(3):351–7, 7.e1. doi:10.1016/j.jpeds.2008.09.017.

[148] Logan JW, 'O'Shea TM, Allred EN, Laughon MM, Bose CL, Dammann O, et al. Early postnatal hypotension and developmental delay at 24 months of age among extremely low gestational age newborns. Arch Dis Child Fetal Neonatal Ed. 2011;96(5):F321–8. Doi:10.1136/adc.2010.183335.

[149] Bishara N, Ohls RK. Current controversies in the management of the anemia of prematurity. Semin Perinatol. 2009;33(1):29–34. Doi:10.1053/j.semperi.2008.10.006.

[150] Whyte RK. Neurodevelopmental outcome of extremely low-birth-weight infants randomly assigned to restrictive or liberal hemoglobin thresholds for blood transfusion. Semin Perinatol. 2012;36(4):290–3. Doi:10.1053/j.semperi.2012.04.010.

[151] Kirpalani H, Whyte RK, Andersen C, Asztalos EV, Heddle N, Blajchman MA, et al. The Premature Infants in Need of Transfusion (PINT) study: a randomized, controlled trial

of a restrictive (low) versus liberal (high) transfusion threshold for extremely low birth weight infants. J Pediatr. 2006;149(3):301–7.

[152] Backes CH, Rivera BK, Haque U, Bridge JA, Smith CV, Hutchon DJ, et al. Placental transfusion strategies in very preterm neonates: a systematic review and meta-analysis. Obstet Gynecol. 2014;124(1):47–56. Doi:10.1097/AOG.0000000000000324.

[153] Committee on Obstetric Practice, American College of Obstetricians and Gynecologists. Committee Opinion No.543: Timing of umbilical cord clamping after birth. Obstet Gynecol. 2012;120(6):1522–6. Doi:10.1097/01.AOG.0000423817.47165.48.

[154] Rabe H, Diaz-Rossello JL, Duley L, Dowswell T. Effect of timing of umbilical cord clamping and other strategies to influence placental transfusion at preterm birth on maternal and infant outcomes. Cochrane Database Syst Rev. 2012;8:CD003248. Doi: 10.1002/14651858.CD003248.pub3.

[155] Rabe H, Jewison A, Alvarez RF, Crook D, Stilton D, Bradley R, et al. Milking compared with delayed cord clamping to increase placental transfusion in preterm neonates: a randomized controlled trial. Obstet Gynecol. 2011;117(2 Pt 1):205–11. Doi:10.1097/AOG.0b013e3181fe46ff.

[156] Aladangady N, McHugh S, Aitchison TC, Wardrop CA, Holland BM. 'Infants' blood volume in a controlled trial of placental transfusion at preterm delivery. Pediatrics. 2006;117(1):93–8.

[157] Aher SM, Ohlsson A. Late erythropoietin for preventing red blood cell transfusion in preterm and/or low birth weight infants. Cochrane Database Syst Rev. 2014;4:CD004868. Doi:10.1002/14651858.CD004868.pub4.

[158] Ohls RK, Kamath-Rayne BD, Christensen RD, Wiedmeier SE, Rosenberg A, Fuller J, et al. Cognitive outcomes of preterm infants randomized to darbepoetin, erythropoietin, or placebo. Pediatrics. 2014;133(6):1023–30. Doi:10.1542/peds.2013-4307.

[159] Benitz WE, Committee on Fetus and Newborn. Patent ductus arteriosus in preterm infants. Pediatrics. 2016;137(1):1–6. Doi:10.1542/peds.2015-3730.

[160] Fanaroff AA, Stoll BJ, Wright LL, Carlo WA, Ehrenkranz RA, Stark AR, et al. Trends in neonatal morbidity and mortality for very low birthweight infants. Am J Obstet Gynecol. 2007;196(2):147.e1–8.

[161] Ohlsson A, Walia R, Shah SS. Ibuprofen for the treatment of patent ductus arteriosus in preterm or low birth weight (or both) infants. Cochrane Database Syst Rev. 2015;2:CD003481. Doi:10.1002/14651858.CD003481.pub6.

[162] Herrera C, Holberton J, Davis P. Prolonged versus short course of indomethacin for the treatment of patent ductus arteriosus in preterm infants. Cochrane Database Syst Rev. 2007;(2):CD003480.

[163] Neumann R, Schulzke SM, Bührer C. Oral ibuprofen versus intravenous ibuprofen or intravenous indomethacin for the treatment of patent ductus arteriosus in preterm

infants: a systematic review and meta-analysis. Neonatology. 2012;102(1):9–15. Doi: 10.1159/000335332.

[164] Malviya MN, Ohlsson A, Shah SS. Surgical versus medical treatment with cyclooxygenase inhibitors for symptomatic patent ductus arteriosus in preterm infants. Cochrane Database Syst Rev. 2013;3:CD003951. Doi:10.1002/14651858.CD003951.pub3.

[165] Fowlie PW, Davis PG, McGuire W. Prophylactic intravenous indomethacin for preventing mortality and morbidity in preterm infants. Cochrane Database Syst Rev. 2010;(7):CD000174. Doi:10.1002/14651858.CD000174.pub2.

[166] Goùrnay V, Roze JC, Kuster A, Daoud P, Cambonie G, Hascoet JM, et al. Prophylactic ibuprofen versus placebo in very premature infants: a randomised, double-blind, placebo-controlled trial. Lancet. 2004;364(9449):1939–44.

[167] Van Overmeire B, Allegaert K, Casaer A, Debauche C, Decaluwé W, Jespers A, et al. Prophylactic ibuprofen in premature infants: a multicentre, randomised, double-blind, placebo-controlled trial. Lancet. 2004;364(9449):1945–9.

[168] Abu-Shaweesh JM, Martin RJ. Neonatal apnea: 'what's new? Pediatr Pulmonol. 2008;43(10):937–44. Doi:10.1002/ppul.20832.

[169] Eichenwald EC, Committee on Fetus and Newborn. Apnea of prematurity. Pediatrics. 2016;137(1):1–7. Doi:10.1542/peds.2015-3757.

[170] Schmidt B, Roberts RS, Davis P, Doyle LW, Barrington KJ, Ohlsson A, et al. Caffeine therapy for apnea of prematurity. N Engl J Med. 2006;354(20):2112–21.

[171] Davis PG, Schmidt B, Roberts RS, Doyle LW, Asztalos E, Haslam R, et al. Caffeine for apnea of prematurity trial: benefits may vary in subgroups. J Pediatr. 2010;156(3):382–7. Doi:10.1016/j.jpeds.2009.09.069.

[172] Lodha A, Seshia M, McMillan DD, Barrington K, Yang J, Lee SK, et al. Association of early caffeine administration and neonatal outcomes in very preterm neonates. JAMA Pediatr. 2015;169(1):33–8. Doi:10.1001/jamapediatrics.2014.2223.

[173] Henderson-Smart DJ, Davis PG. Prophylactic methylxanthines for endotracheal extubation in preterm infants. Cochrane Database Syst Rev. 2010;(12):CD000139. Doi: 10.1002/14651858.CD000139.pub2.

[174] Schmidt B, Roberts RS, Davis P, Doyle LW, Barrington KJ, Ohlsson A, et al. Long-term effects of caffeine therapy for apnea of prematurity. N Engl J Med. 2007;357(19):1893–902.

[175] Schmidt B, Anderson PJ, Doyle LW, Dewey D, Grunau RE, Asztalos EV, et al. Survival without disability to age 5 years after neonatal caffeine therapy for apnea of prematurity. JAMA. 2012;307(3):275–82. Doi:10.1001/jama.2011.2024.

[176] Doyle LW, Schmidt B, Anderson PJ, Davis PG, Moddemann D, Grunau RE, et al. Reduction in developmental coordination disorder with neonatal caffeine therapy. J Pediatr. 2014;165(2):356–9.e2. doi:10.1016/j.jpeds.2014.04.016.

[177] Watterberg KL, American Academy of Pediatrics. Committee on Fetus and Newborn. Policy statement—postnatal corticosteroids to prevent or treat bronchopulmonary dysplasia. Pediatrics. 2010;126(4):800–8. Doi:10.1542/peds.2010-1534.

[178] Tanney K, Davis J, Halliday HL, Sweet DG. Extremely low-dose dexamethasone to facilitate extubation in mechanically ventilated preterm babies. Neonatology. 2011;100(3):285–9. Doi:10.1159/000326273.

[179] Hitzert MM, Benders MJ, Roescher AM, van Bel F, de Vries LS, Bos AF. Hydrocortisone vs. dexamethasone treatment for bronchopulmonary dysplasia and their effects on general movements in preterm infants. Pediatr Res. 2012;71(1):100–6. Doi:10.1038/pr.2011.15.